Sandra Blöthner

Somatic alterations in critical genes in malignant melanoma

Sandra Blöthner

Somatic alterations in critical genes in malignant melanoma

Effect on global gene expression

Südwestdeutscher Verlag für Hochschulschriften

Impressum/Imprint (nur für Deutschland/ only for Germany)
Bibliografische Information der Deutschen Nationalbibliothek: Die Deutsche Nationalbibliothek verzeichnet diese Publikation in der Deutschen Nationalbibliografie; detaillierte bibliografische Daten sind im Internet über http://dnb.d-nb.de abrufbar.
Alle in diesem Buch genannten Marken und Produktnamen unterliegen warenzeichen-, marken- oder patentrechtlichem Schutz bzw. sind Warenzeichen oder eingetragene Warenzeichen der jeweiligen Inhaber. Die Wiedergabe von Marken, Produktnamen, Gebrauchsnamen, Handelsnamen, Warenbezeichnungen u.s.w. in diesem Werk berechtigt auch ohne besondere Kennzeichnung nicht zu der Annahme, dass solche Namen im Sinne der Warenzeichen- und Markenschutzgesetzgebung als frei zu betrachten wären und daher von jedermann benutzt werden dürften.

Verlag: Südwestdeutscher Verlag für Hochschulschriften Aktiengesellschaft & Co. KG
Dudweiler Landstr. 99, 66123 Saarbrücken, Deutschland
Telefon +49 681 37 20 271-1, Telefax +49 681 37 20 271-0, Email: info@svh-verlag.de
Zugl.: Heidelberg, Ruprecht-Karls-Universität, Diss., 2006

Herstellung in Deutschland:
Schaltungsdienst Lange o.H.G., Berlin
Books on Demand GmbH, Norderstedt
Reha GmbH, Saarbrücken
Amazon Distribution GmbH, Leipzig
ISBN: 978-3-8381-0422-5

Imprint (only for USA, GB)
Bibliographic information published by the Deutsche Nationalbibliothek: The Deutsche Nationalbibliothek lists this publication in the Deutsche Nationalbibliografie; detailed bibliographic data are available in the Internet at http://dnb.d-nb.de.
Any brand names and product names mentioned in this book are subject to trademark, brand or patent protection and are trademarks or registered trademarks of their respective holders. The use of brand names, product names, common names, trade names, product descriptions etc. even without a particular marking in this works is in no way to be construed to mean that such names may be regarded as unrestricted in respect of trademark and brand protection legislation and could thus be used by anyone.

Publisher:
Südwestdeutscher Verlag für Hochschulschriften Aktiengesellschaft & Co. KG
Dudweiler Landstr. 99, 66123 Saarbrücken, Germany
Phone +49 681 37 20 271-1, Fax +49 681 37 20 271-0, Email: info@svh-verlag.de

Copyright © 2009 by the author and Südwestdeutscher Verlag für Hochschulschriften Aktiengesellschaft & Co. KG and licensors
All rights reserved. Saarbrücken 2009

Printed in the U.S.A.
Printed in the U.K. by (see last page)
ISBN: 978-3-8381-0422-5

„Unsere Wünsche sind die Vorboten der Fähigkeiten, die in uns liegen."

Johann Wolfgang von Goethe
deutscher Dichter (1749 - 1832)

To my Family

CONTENTS

ABBREVIATIONS

1. INTRODUCTION 9
   1.1. CUTANEOUS MALIGNANT MELANOMA 9
      1.1.1. Incidence 9
      1.1.2. Risk Factors 9
      1.1.3. Melanoma Progression 11
      1.1.4. Types of Melanoma 12
      1.1.5. Melanoma Classification and Prognosis 12
   1.2. GENETICS OF MELANOMA 15
      1.2.1. The *CDKN2A* gene locus 15
      1.2.2. Alterations of the *CDKN2A* gene locus in melanoma 19
      1.2.3. The *CDK4* gene 21
      1.2.4. The RAS-RAF-MEK-ERK Pathway 21
   1.3. GLOBAL GENE EXPRESSION ANALYSIS USING
        MICROARRAY TECHNOLOGY 27
      1.3.1. Microarray technology and human cancers 27
      1.3.2. Gene expression profiling of malignant melanoma 27

2. AIMS OF THE STUDY 29

3. MATERIALS AND METHODS 30
   3.1. MELANOMA CELL LINES 30
      3.1.1. Cell lines and cell culture 30
      3.1.2. Isolation of DNA and RNA 31
      3.1.3. DNA sequencing 32
      3.1.4. Global gene expression in melanoma cells 34
   3.2. MELANOCYTIC NEVI 37
      3.2.1. Origin/Subjects 37
      3.2.2. Isolation of DNA and RNA 38
      3.2.3. Mutation detection 39
      3.2.4. Global gene expression in melanocytic nevi 39
   3.3. MICROARRAY DATA ANALYSIS 43
      3.3.1. Image Analysis 43
      3.3.2. GeneChip Operating Software (GCOS) 43
      3.3.3. Significance Analysis of Microarrays (SAM) 44
      3.3.4. GeneCluster2.0 44

   3.3.5. Identification of differentially expressed genes 45

  3.4. QUANTITATIVE REAL-TIME PCR 46

   3.4.1. Validation of microarray expression results 46
   3.4.2. Determination of expression levels of B-RAF, N-RAS
     and CDKN2A in melanoma cell lines 47
   3.4.3. Determination of the AKAP9 – B-RAF fusion transcript
     in melanoma cell lines 48

4. RESULTS 50

  4.1. Mutations in the *B-RAF* and *N-RAS* genes and homozygous deletions
    of the *CDKN2A* gene locus in melanoma cell lines 50
  4.2. Levels of B-RAF, N-RAS and CDKN2A gene expression and
    correlation with mutations 53
  4.3. The AKAP9 – B-RAF fusion transcript in melanoma cell lines 54
  4.4. Effect of V600E *B-RAF* and Q61R *N-RAS* mutations on
    global gene expression in melanoma cell lines 55
  4.5. Differences in global gene expression in melanoma cell lines with and
    without homozygous deletions of the *CDKN2A* locus genes 64
  4.6. Effect of the V600E *B-RAF* mutation on global gene expression in
    melanocytic nevi 71

5. DISCUSSION 78

  5.1. Mutations in the *B-RAF* and *N-RAS* genes and alterations of the
    CDKN2A gene locus in melanoma cell lines 78
  5.2. Expression of B-RAF, N-RAS and CDKN2A and correlation with
    mutations in melanoma cell lines 80
  5.3. Absence of the AKAP9 – B-RAF fusion transcript in melanoma cell lines 80
  5.4. Effects of common genetic alterations on gene expression in
    melanoma cell lines and melanocytic nevi 82
   5.4.1. *Effect of B-RAF V600E and N-RAS Q61R mutations*
     on global gene expression in melanoma cell lines 82
   5.4.2. *Effect of homozygous deletion of the CDKN2A locus genes*
     on global gene expression in melanoma cell lines 85
   5.4.3. *Effect of the B-RAF V600E mutation on global gene*
     expression in melanocytic nevi 88

6. SUMMARY 91

7. REFERENCES 92

8. APPENDIX 109

9. OWN PUBLICATIONS 130

10. ACKNOWLEDGEMENTS 131

ABBREVIATIONS

AKAP9	A-kinase anchor protein 9
ARF	Alternate reading frame
aRNA	amplified RNA
bp	Base pairs
B-RAF	V-raf murine sarcoma viral oncogene homolog B1
cAMP	cyclic adenosine monophosphate
CDKN2A	Cyclin-dependend kinase inhibitor 2A
CDK4/6	Cyclin-dependend kinase 4/6
cDNA	complementary DNA
DMT	Data Mining Tool
dNTP	Deoxyribonucleotide triphosphate
DTT	Dithiothreitol
FDR	False discovery rate
GCOS	GeneChip Operating Software
GDP	Guanosine diphosphate
GTP	Guanosine triphosphate
ERK1/2	Mitogen-activated protein kinase 3/1
MAPK	Mitogen-activated protein kinase
MEK1/2	Mitogen-activated kinase kinase 1/2
ml	Millilitre
mM	Millimolar
µl	Microlitre
ng	Nanogram
N-RAS	Neuroblastoma ras viral oncogene homolog
OD	Optical density
OR	Odds ratio
PCR	Polymerase chain reaction
RGP	Radial growth phase
rpm	Rounds per minute
SAM	Significance Analysis of Microarrays
U	Unit
UV	Ultraviolet
VGP	Vertical growth phase

1. INTRODUCTION

1.1. CUTANEOUS MALIGNANT MELANOMA

1.1.1. Incidence

Melanoma is the most aggressive and potentially lethal skin tumour. It originates in pigment-producing melanocytes that are found in the basal layer of the epidermis and in the eye (1). The number of melanoma cases and deaths worldwide has increased faster than many other cancers though of late the trend has stabilised (2-4). The annual increase in incidence rates has been 3–7% per year for white-skinned Caucasian populations (5, 6). Estimates suggested a doubling of melanoma incidence every 10-20 years (7). Highest annual incidence rates are found in Australia and New Zealand with about 56 cases per 100 000 inhabitants with no statistically significant differences between males and females (2, 8). Other countries with high melanoma incidence rates are USA and Canada (9, 10). In Europe, highest incidence rates have been reported in Scandinavia with about 15 cases per 100 000 inhabitants (11, 12). In Germany, incidence rate is about 10-12 cases per 100 000 inhabitants (11). Lowest incidence rates in Europe are reported in Mediterranean countries with about 5–7 cases per 100 000 inhabitants (11, 13, 14). The north-south gradient in melanoma incidence in Europe has been explained by the differences in skin pigmentation between the populations (11). At global level, lowest annual incidence rates are found in Asian countries with rates near 0.5 cases per 100 000 inhabitants (15, 16). Melanoma is rare in individuals below 20 years of age and frequent in young and middle aged adults (6, 17, 18).

1.1.2. Risk Factors

An individual´s risk of developing melanoma depends on two sets of factors: a) host related factors such as pigmentation characteristics and skin reaction to sunlight; and b) environmental factors (Table 1) (19-21). The only known environmental risk factor is exposure to ultraviolet (UV) light. Epidemiological evidence suggests that high-intensity intermittent sun exposure is the key factor in induction of the majority of melanomas (22, 23). The risk of melanoma is higher in fair-skinned people, especially those with blonde or red hair who sunburn and freckle easily, than in people with darker complexions (24). In addition to UV exposure, age at exposure is an important determinant of the risk of melanoma. Several studies have suggested a strong link between sunburn in childhood and development of melanocytic neoplasia later in life (25). High sun exposure during adult life constitutes a significant risk factor for melanoma only if there had been substantial sun exposure during childhood (26).

Table 1. Melanoma risk factors.

Constitutional predisposition
Fair skin and hair colour
Number of benign nevi (moles)
Freckles
Presence of three or more atypical nevi
Propensity to burn in the sun rather than tan
Prior therapy with psoralen and ultraviolet (UV) A light
History of solar keratoses, squamous cell carcinoma, or xeroderma pigmentosum
Family history of dysplastic nevi or melanoma

Risk behaviours
History of three or more episodes of sunburn, especially during childhood
Episodic excessive sunlight exposure (e.g., recreational tanning)
Long term continuous sunlight exposure (e.g., outdoor workers)
UV exposure at tanning salons

Environmental factors
Stratospheric ozone depletion, latitudes closer to equator (e.g., higher UV radiation)

The presence of atypical or dysplastic melanocytic nevi are major markers for melanoma risk across all continents, both in high risk families and in the general population (27, 28). Also the presence of multiple, non-dysplastic moles points to increased melanoma risk (29, 30). Genetic predisposition in families is in part attributed to two melanoma susceptibility genes. Germline alterations in the major melanoma susceptibility gene, *CDKN2A* on chromosome 9p21, occur in 25-40% of melanoma families (31, 32). The *CDK4* oncogene on chromosome 12q14 is considered to be another melanoma susceptibility gene. However, to date, worldwide only in four families melanoma-prone kindreds have been reported to carry mutations in *CDK4* (33-35).

1.1.3. Melanoma Progression

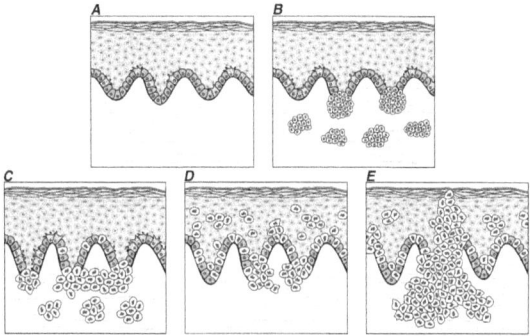

Figure 1. Stages of melanoma progression. A) Normal skin, B) Benign proliferation of melanocytes, C) Melanocyte dysplasia, D) *In situ* melanoma (RGP), E) Malignant melanoma (VGP). [reprinted by permission from Genes & Development (Sherr, 13:1501-12) Copyright (2001) Cold Spring Harbor Laboratory Press].

Melanoma is typically the final stage of a multi-stage evolution in a series of melanocytic lesions. Approximately 20-30% of melanomas arise from pre-existing common nevi or moles; however, the majority of melanomas arise *de novo* (36, 37). Melanocytic nevi can be present at birth (congenital) or arise during an individual´s lifetime. Nevi are classified as junctional (lesional cells at the epidermal-dermal interface), intradermal (cells located in the dermis), or compound (cells present in both epidermis or junction and dermis) (38). Dysplastic or atypical nevi also bear junctional architecture but, unlike other nevi, show nuclear atypia (39). The first transition in melanomagenesis appears to be the conversion of a normal melanocyte into a benign and then dysplastic nevus (atypical mole) (40, 41). In normal skin, dendritic melanocytes are evenly distributed throughout the basal layer of the skin (Figure 1A). A benign nevus appears as an aggregation of non-dendritic melanocytes, that have stopped growing due to cellular senescence (41, 42) (Figure 1B). In dysplastic nevi, the aggregates appear irregular and consist of large atypical melanocytes (Figure 1C). Dysplastic nevi can progress to an *in situ* melanoma, which grows laterally and is mostly confined to the epidermis, called the radial growth phase (RGP) (Figure 1D). RGP melanoma can be treated effectively by surgical resection with a low risk of relapse or metastasis. If left untreated the melanoma can progress to the vertical growth phase (VGP), which is associated with invasion of the melanoma cells into the dermis and the acquisition of metastatic potential (Figure 1E)(43, 44). Metastatic melanomas are aggressive lesions with ability to spread to many peripheral organs such as the brain, liver, lungs and heart and at the advanced stage, there are no effective treatments (45).

1.1.4. Types of Melanoma

Melanoma types are determined by their growth and microscopic characteristics and physical history. The American Joint Committee on Cancer (AJCC) has identified five different forms of extraocular melanoma: superficial spreading melanoma (SSM), nodular malignant melanoma (NM), lentigo maligna melanoma (LMM), acral-lentiginous melanoma (ALM), and mucosal lentiginous melanoma (MLM). SSM is the most common form of cutaneous melanoma, accounting for approximately 70% of all melanomas. SSM mostly occurs on the head, neck, and trunk in men and on the extremities in women. NM is the second most common melanoma, comprising 10–15% of all cutaneous melanomas. NM occurs on any body surface area but is most commonly diagnosed on the trunk of men. NM does not have a radial growth phase and is associated with rapid evolution to vertical growth and invasion of the dermis; therefore it is thought to be biologically more aggressive than SSM. LMM and ALM constitute approximately 5-10% of all melanomas and are the least common types of melanoma. LMM almost always appears on sun-exposed areas of the head and neck of elderly people. ALM occurs on the palms, soles and nail beds. Although similar in clinical appearance to LMM, ALM is a biologically much more aggressive lesion with a short evolution to the vertical growth phase. MLM accounts for approximately 3% of the melanomas diagnosed annually. This lesion develops from the mucosal epithelium that lines the respiratory, gastrointestinal, and genitourinary systems and is usually diagnosed in patients of advanced age. Melanoma can also occur in the eye (ocular melanoma) and like other types of melanoma it can be treated and cured if detected early. Signs of ocular melanoma are spots on the iris, distortion of the pupil and new blood vessels appearing in the eye.

1.1.5. Melanoma Classification and Prognosis

Melanomas are classified according to the Breslow system and the Clark´s system (Figure 2). The Breslow system measures precisely the thickness of the tumour from the skin surface (i.e. epidermis) to its deepest point on invasion as seen under the microscope. The thicker the tumour, the poorer is the prognosis. The Clark's level of invasion refers to the extent of penetration of the tumour into the skin:

- **Level 1** is known as in-situ melanoma in which the cancer cells are limited to the upper most layer of the skin (i.e. the epidermis) and as such it has no potential to spread and is therefore 100% curable.

- **Levels II, III and IV** refer to an increasing degree of invasion of melanoma cells into the true skin (i.e. the dermis). Once the cancer cells have invaded the fat layer, it is referred to as **Level V**. The deeper the penetration of the cancer into the skin, the poorer the prognosis.

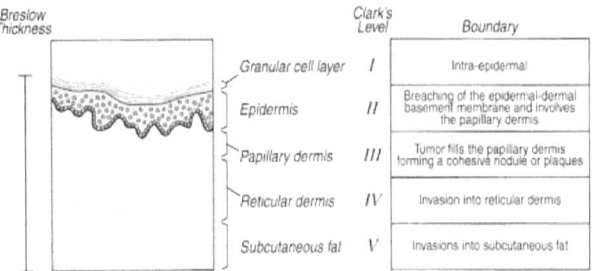

Figure 2. Pathological classification of melanoma according to Breslow thickness and Clark's classification system. [reprinted by permission from Genes & Development (Chin *et al.*, 12:3467-81) Copyright (2001) Cold Spring Harbor Laboratory Press].

In recent years, physicians have adopted a more distinguishable method of classification which incorporates information about the level of invasion, or tumour thickness in addition to the extent of spread to other sites. This system is known as the AJCC/TNM system (46, 47):

- **Stage IA**- Primary melanoma less than or equal to 0.75 mm thick and/or Clark's level II, localized disease to the original tumour site, with no evidence of spread.
- **Stage IB**- Primary melanoma 0.76 to 1.5 mm thick and/or Clark's level III. No sign of tumours in the lymph nodes or other organs.
- **Stage IIA**- Primary melanoma 1.51 to 4 mm thick and/or Clark's level IV; no signs of tumours in the lymph nodes or any other organs.
- **Stage IIB**- Primary melanoma greater than 4 mm thick and/or Clark's level V; no signs of tumours on the lymph nodes or any other organs.
- **Stage III**- Spread to the regional lymph nodes and/or in-transit metastatic tumours.
- **Stage IV**- Distant metastasis. Spread to other organs in the body.

The most important prognostic factor is the disease stage at diagnosis, represented by Clark´s level and Breslow´s thickness (48). Other variables that have prognostic value for the patient´s survival include patient´s age at diagnosis, sex, anatomic location of the primary tumour, size, and histopathologic type (48-51). It has been summarised that tumour thickness and ulceration are highly predictive of survival (52). The prognosis of thin, non-ulcerated tumours is excellent (53).

The mitotic rate per mm^2 and the presence or absence of lymphatic or blood vessel invasion are also relevant to prognosis (51, 54, 55). Women with melanoma show a better prognosis than men (49, 56). Both male and female patients with melanomas of the extremities have a better survival rate than patients with melanomas of the head and neck; patients with melanomas of the trunk are associated with worst prognosis (57, 58). Melanoma is highly curable by surgical excision, if diagnosed at an early stage. Late-stage melanoma with distant metastatic spread shows a very poor prognosis; with a low response rate to conventional chemotherapy (59). Melanoma has the ability to spread to almost any organ site. The median survival is 7-12 months for patients with one metastatic site but only 2-8 months for patients with multiple metastatic sites (50, 60).

1.2. GENETICS OF MELANOMA

1.2.1. The CDKN2A gene locus

The tumour suppressor p16^{INK4A} (henceforth called p16) was identified through two independend lines of research. In cell biology experiments, it was detected through its interaction with CDK4 in a yeast two-hybrid screen (61). Simultaneously, the gene *CDKN2A (MTS1)* was mapped to the frequently altered chromosome 9p21 locus by positional cloning (62, 63). The p16 protein consists of 156 amino acids encoded by three exons.

Subsequent to the discovery of p16, a second transcript arising from the *CDKN2A* locus was discovered, which comprised of an alternate exon 1β located about 20 kb upstream of the regular exon 1α. Exon 1β splices with exons 2 and 3 to transcribe p14^{ARF} (henceforth called ARF) from a separate promoter (*p19^{ARF}* in the mouse). The ARF transcript is translated in an alternate reading frame (Figure 3). The human ARF protein consists of 132 amino acids. The two proteins, p16 and ARF, encoded from a partially shared genomic sequence are structurally unrelated. Incidentally, both function as cell cycle inhibitors (64, 65). P16 functions in the retinoblastoma pathway and ARF in the p53 pathway of cell cycle regulation. Adjacent to the *CDKN2A*, two exons of *CDKN2B* encode p15^{INK4B}. P15^{INK4B} is homologous and functionally similar to p16^{INK4A} (Figure 3)(66, 67).

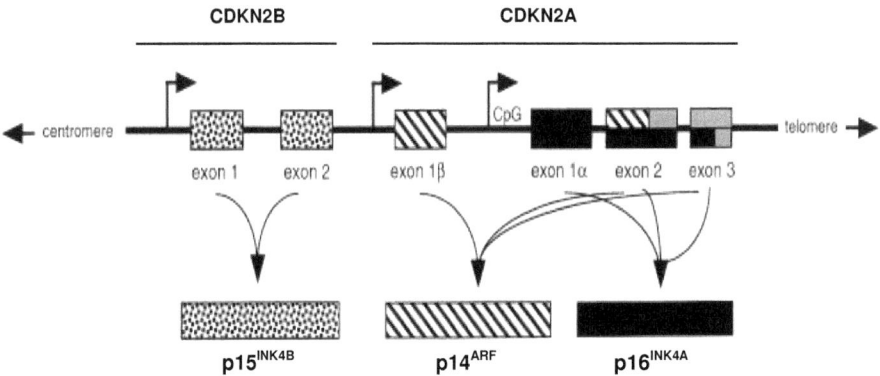

Figure 3. Genomic organisation of the *CDKN2A* and *CDKN2B* gene loci on chromosome 9p21 and the transcripts arising from these loci.

The *CDKN2A* gene locus represents a unique structure in the mammalian genome. Overlapping gene structures are common in viral and bacterial genomes. In the small-sized viral genomes, this structure type represents an important mechanism to maximize the usage of the coding sequence (65). The unique genomic organization of the *CDKN2A* gene locus may explain why p16/ARF is a frequent target of inactivation in tumourigenesis. A single genetic hit results in the simultaneous disruption of two key anti-oncogenic mechanisms.

p16 and the retinoblastoma pathway
In hypophosphorylated state, retinoblastoma (Rb) binds to E2F transcription factors, which are necessary for the progression of the cell cycle from G1 to S phase (68, 69). The enzymatic complex of CDK4/6 and cyclin D positively regulates the cell cycle by phosphorylating Rb. However, p16 disrupts the kinase complex of CDK4/6 and cyclin D by binding to CDK4. It inhibits the phosphorylation of Rb and therefore negatively regulates cell cycle progression (Figure 4) (70). Ankyrin-like repeats in the protein sequence motif of p16 are involved in binding to CDK4 (61, 71).

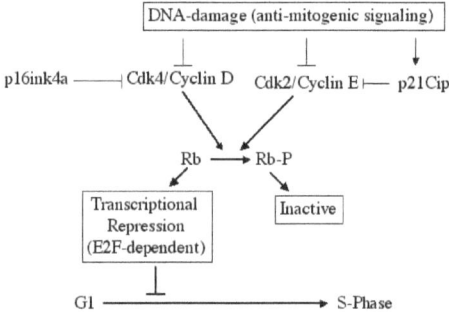

Figure 4. p16 and the Rb pathway. P16 binds directly to CDK4 to disrupt the complex with cyclin D. Inhibition of the cyclin D-CDK4/6 complex results in Rb hypophosphorylation, which in turn represses E2F-dependent gene expression and blocks G_1/S cell cycle progression.

ARF and the p53 pathway
The ARF protein acts as a cell cycle inhibitor by antagonising MDM2-mediated degradation of p53, thereby stabilising this tumour suppressor protein (Figure 5) (72, 73). The exact mechanism whereby ARF stabilises p53 is not entirely clear. Three models for the mechanism of p53 stabilisation by ARF have been proposed (74). One model suggests that ARF localises to the nucleolus and sequesters MDM2 to that compartment, resulting in release of p53 from MDM2

inhibition (75, 76). Another proposed mechanism is the formation of ternary complexes of ARF, MDM2 and p53 in the nucleoplasm, which prevents nuclear export of both MDM2 and p53 (77). A third possible mechanism is that ARF need not to relocate MDM2 to the nucleolus for proper function; but rather only inhibits the E3-ligase activity of MDM2 to stabilise p53 (78, 79).

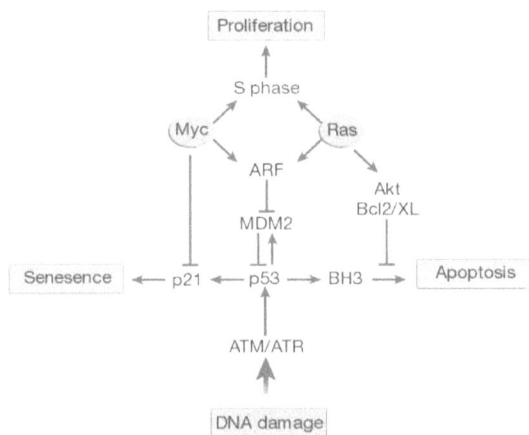

Figure 5. ARF and the p53 pathway. DNA damage or oncogenic signals like MYC or RAS activate the p53 pathway, resulting in induction of apoptosis or senescence. The ARF protein acts as a cell cycle inhibitor by antagonising MDM2-mediated degradation of p53. [reprinted by permission from Nature Reviews (Lowe et al., 432:307-15) Copyright (2004) Nature Publishing Group]

Expression of c-myc, E2F, mutated RAS or loss of Rb induces ARF (80-83). This response to oncogene expression depends on cellular context; RAS potently induces ARF in murine, but not human, cells (83-85). In murine embryonic fibroblasts (MEFs), ARF expression correlates with the onset of senescence, and cells lacking ARF do not senesce in culture (86, 87). In contrast, ARF does not play a major role in the replicative senescence of human cells (88, 89). Recently, interactions of ARF with SUMO-E2, AP-1 dimers, BCL6, p63, DP1 and nucleophosmin (NPM)/B23 have been reported (90-95). By degradation of B23, ARF decreases the processing of ribosomal RNA, thereby limiting cell growth and inducing cell cycle arrest (95, 96). Repressor molecules such as Twist, TBX2, and Pokemon have been shown to inhibit ARF expression (97-99).

Cdkn2a knockout studies

The major support for the tumour suppressor function of the *CDKN2A* gene locus came from knockout studies. The construction of different types of knockout mice provided comparisons of *p16*- and *Arf*-null phenotypes respectively. In the first *Cdkn2a* knockout mice exon 2 was ablated, resulting in inactivation of both the *p16* and *Arf* transcripts (100). These animals did not develop melanoma, but were prone to the development of other tumours, like fibrosarcomas and lymphomas. To assess the effects of deleting the *Arf* transcript alone, exon 1β of the *Cdkn2a* locus was knocked out in mice (86). The animals expressed a similar phenotype to the *p16/Arf*-null mice, suggesting that inactivation of *Arf*, rather than *p16*, may be responsible for the tumour susceptibility phenotype in the first model. Mice with deletion of one copy of *Arf* combined with complete inactivation of *p16* developed melanomas with very high penetrance, compared to *p16* knockout mice that retained both *Arf* alleles. *Arf* appears to be haploinsufficient in this context, suggesting cooperation between the p16 and Arf pathways in melanoma development (101). Crossing of *p16/Arf*-null mice with mice overexpressing oncogenic *H-ras* (Tyr-*H-ras* transgenic mice) resulted in offspring, which developed cutaneous malignant melanoma spontaneously with a high penetrance (102). These data support the hypothesis, that further genetic events in addition to *CDKN2A* inactivation are required for melanocyte tumourigenesis. Two groups later generated specific, "pure" p16 knockout mice. In one model (designated Ink4a$^{*/*}$), a stop signal at codon 101 in exon 2 was introduced, producing a truncated and unstable p16 protein (101). In the other type (termed Ink4a$^{\Delta exon1\alpha}$), exon 1α was deleted (84). In both knockouts the expression of *Arf* was unaffected. The "pure" *p16*-null mice had a lower frequency of spontaneous tumour development than the *Arf*-null mice. Importantly, like mice with deletion of one copy of *Arf* and *p16* inactivation, the "pure" *p16*-null mice were susceptible to spontaneous melanoma development, albeit at lower frequency. Altogether, the knockout studies indicate that both genes, *p16* and *Arf*, function as tumour suppressors in mice. Significantly, both types of "pure" *p16* knockout mice developed melanoma, which was detected neither in *p16/Arf*-null mice nor in *Arf*-null mice.

Data from other non-murine model systems also support the notion that p16 functions as a tumour suppressor gene. Primary melanomas and osteosarcoma cell lines from canines harbor frequent *p16* inactivation (103, 104). Rat carcinogen models show a high incidence of *p16* promoter methylation and *p16/Arf* deletion (105, 106). Strains of the fish Xiphophorus are prone to melanoma. Susceptibility in this species maps to the *DIFF* locus, which is tightly linked to the Xiphophorus *INK4A* locus (107).

1.2.2. Alterations of the CDKN2A gene locus in melanoma

Germline alterations

The *CDKN2A* has been identified as a high penetrance melanoma susceptibility gene. One of the most significant risk factors for melanoma is a family history of the disease. It is estimated that ~10% of melanoma cases report a first- or second-degree relative with melanoma. Epidemiological studies suggest that the estimated genetic component in malignant melanoma is ~18% (108, 109). Analysis of familial cancer risk of melanoma has shown a risk of ~2.5 for an offspring when a parent had melanoma (110). Around 50% of the melanoma-prone kindreds show genetic linkage to markers within the 9p21 region, and of those, ~40% carried germline mutations in *CDKN2A* (32, 35, 111). Data from families studied world-wide indicate that the frequency of *CDKN2A* mutations increases with i) the number of melanoma cases in the family, ii) the presence of individuals with multiple melanomas and iii) an age at diagnosis < 50 years (112). In addition to melanoma, the mutation carriers are at an increased risk of pancreatic cancer. Several studies have reported the occurrence of pancreatic cancer in *CDKN2A* mutation-positive melanoma families (113, 114).

Recently, *ARF* mutations have been suggested to predispose to melanoma, as well as to nervous system tumours (NSTs) (115, 116). This combination of tumours has been proposed as a discrete syndrome by several investigators (117, 118). A specific germline deletion of *ARF* in the absence of concomitant loss of *p16* was found in a family segregating melanomas and NSTs (119). It has been concluded that exon 1β alone is sufficient for ARF function (120). A deletion of exon 1β of *ARF* was found in a family where mother and daughter had melanoma (121). A germline 16 bp insertion in exon 1β was detected in a patient with multiple melanomas but without a family history of the disease (122). Exon 1β mutations that do not alter p16 function have been reported in kindreds with familial melanoma and astrocytoma (119, 122). A cluster of five different germline mutations at the *ARF* exon 1β splice donor site was recently identified in melanoma pedigrees; three of the variants resulted in aberrant splicing of the ARF mRNA (123).

CDKN2A alterations in sporadic melanoma

The *CDKN2A (p16)* gene is involved in the development of sporadic melanoma. Monoallelic deletion of the *CDKN2A* gene locus is found in ~50% of primary tumours and nearly all melanoma cell lines (124-126). However, some reports have not found frequent alterations, thereby the role of *CDKN2A (p16)* in sporadic melanoma appears inconsistent (127, 128). Genetic alterations of *p16* involved in sporadic melanoma are point mutations (0-26%), promoter methylation (0-10%), and homozygous deletions (5-25%) (129). Intragenic mutations and hypermethylation of the *p16* promoter appear to be rare (130-132). The low frequency of mutations of *p16* in conjunction with a high frequency of allelic losses at chromosome 9p21 has also been interpreted as an indicator of the presence of other tumour suppressor genes at this locus (126, 133-135). Loss of p16 expression is associated with advanced stages of sporadic melanomas and a high mitotic index, suggesting that loss of p16 is a late event in the progression of sporadic primary melanomas (136, 137). In another report, the degree of p16 expression was related to the histological type of tumour (138). Increased allelic loss at 9p21 correlated also with increased patient age at diagnosis (134). Homozygous deletions affecting p16 are more frequent in melanoma cell lines than in primary tumours, which in part is due to technical constraints in detection of homozygous deletions in tumours (124, 127).

CDKN2A polymorphisms
The *CDKN2A* gene carries several polymorphisms. Two polymorphisms in the 3´untranslated region of the *CDKN2A* gene, C500G and C540T, have been associated with melanoma (139, 140). The C500G change ablates an *MspI*/*Hpa*II restriction site; it has an estimated allele frequency of ~12-15% (141, 142). The C540T change results in the loss of a *Hae*III site; its frequency is estimated of ~20-25% (126, 142). The functional importance of these polymorphisms is not known, but carriers of either of these variants had a significantly shorter progression time from diagnosis of the primary tumour to the appearance of metastasis (143). On the other hand, presence of the C540T polymorphism in multivariate analysis was significantly associated with improved survival in patients with VGP tumours (144).

Several additional polymorphisms of the *CDKN2A* gene are known, that do not alter the amino acid sequence of p16 or which are functionally indistinguishable from the wild-type protein (145, 146). The most extensively documented polymorphism, A148T, has previously been shown to have no effect on p16 protein function (145, 147). However, in a recent study, A148T was associated with an increased risk of development of melanoma (148). Furthermore, in a case-control study the A148T polymorphism was detected in significantly higher proportion in multiple primary melanoma cases compared to healthy controls (149).

Alterations of p16 and ARF in other cancers
Inactivation of p16 by point mutation, homozygous deletion or promoter methylation is seen in approximately one third of human cancers (129, 146, 150). Missense mutations occur in the entire gene, but particularly in the regions that encode helices of the ankyrin repeats (151). Mutations in

the ankyrin repeats of p16 correlate with impaired binding with and inhibition of CDK4 (152). Besides melanoma, other sporadic cancers with documented mutations and homozygous deletions of *CDKN2A* include esophageal and pancreatic carcinoma, leukemia, and head and neck squamous cell carcinoma (126, 153-156). Methylation of *CDKN2A* with associated silenced transcription has been reported in head and neck, lung, brain, colon, gastric, and esophagus and bladder cancers (129, 157-160). Deletions of the *CDKN2A* locus have been frequently found in numerous tumour cell lines (62, 63). Selective deletion of ARF-specific exon 1β has been detected in T cell acute lymphoblastic leukemias, brain lymphomas and melanoma cell lines (115, 161, 162). Promoter methylation of ARF has been reported in colorectal, gastric, esophageal and endometrial cancers, gliomas, and hepatocellular carcinomas (163-167). Thus, selective inactivation of ARF with intact p16 function occurs in some tumour types. Other tumour types, such as glioblastomas, seem to require concomitant inactivation of both genes for tumour formation (150, 168).

1.2.3. The CDK4 gene

Beside *CDKN2A*, the *CDK4* oncogene on chromosome 12q14 is considered to be another melanoma susceptibility gene; however, only four melanoma-prone kindreds have been reported to carry mutations in *CDK4*. All mutations involved codon 24 of the gene. Two families carried a Arg24Cys germline point mutation (33); two other families an Arg24His substitution (34, 35). CDK4 is a key regulator of the cell cycle. Binding to p16 prevents CDK4 from forming a complex with cyclin D, thereby blocking phosphorylation of Rb and cell cycle progression (169). Both types of mutations affect the p16-binding domain of the CDK4 protein, generating an activated oncogene that is resistant to inhibition by p16 (33). Mice with knocked-in Arg24Cys mutation develop pancreatic hyperplasia and are highly susceptible to development of melanoma after carcinogenic exposure to 7,12-dimethylbenz(a)anthracene (DMBA) and 12-0-tetradecanoylphorbol-13-acetate (TPA) (170, 171).

1.2.4. The RAS-RAF-MEK-ERK Pathway

The RAS-RAF-MEK-ERK pathway is a highly conserved signalling pathway and has been found to play an important role in melanocytic neoplasia (172, 173). Activation of this pathway in cutaneous melanocytes has been shown to occur by a variety of mechanisms that include autocrine growth factor stimulation and oncogenic mutations in the *B-RAF* or *N-RAS* genes (173, 174). RAS proteins are small G-proteins that are embedded on the inner surface of the plasma membrane (175). Those proteins are downstream of a variety of transmembrane receptors, and are activated when GDP is converted to GTP. In the active GTP-bound state, RAS activates a number of downstream signalling cascades involved in controlling cell growth and behaviour. Initially, RAS interacts with and activates B-RAF that transduces regulatory signals from RAS to MEK1/2. The signal transducer MEK1/2 phosphorylates ERK1/2, leading to the activation of these kinases, which in turn activate a variety of transcription factors (Figure 6). ERK phosphorylates many substrates, thereby regulating numerous cellular functions, such as gene expression, metabolism and morphology. Both the duration and intensity of ERK activity are important (176). Consequently, ERK signalling plays an important role in determining cellular fate, choosing between diverse responses such as proliferation, differentiation, senescence or survival (177).

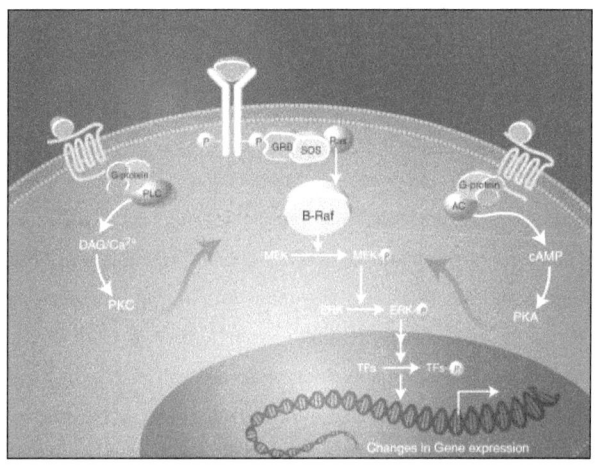

Figure 6. The RAS-RAF-MEK-ERK pathway in melanocyte signal transduction.
[reprinted from Pollock *et al.*, *Cancer Cell*, 2(1):5-7 Copyright (2002), with permission from Elsevier]

In melanocytes, ERK is also activated in the cAMP-dependent signalling cascade as a consequence of α-melanocyte-stimulating hormone and related peptide binding to melanocortin-1 receptor with B-RAF as a key intermediate (178, 179). A major way by which ERK signalling promotes cell cycle progression is through transcriptional upregulation of cyclin D1 (180). Cyclin D1 forms a complex with CDK4/6, which phosphorylates the retinoblastoma protein and allows cells to progress from the G1 to S phase of the cell cycle. Examples of genes that are transcriptionally induced in response to ERK activation include *VEGF*, a positive regulator of angiogenesis, and *MMP-1*, a collagenase involved in degradation of the extracellular matrix (181, 182). Sustained

ERK activation has also been shown to induce expression of β3-integrin in certain cell types (183). Proteins such as VEGF, MMP-1 and β3-integrin are believed to play crucial roles in RAS-mediated tumour cell invasion and metastasis (184).

The RAF genes

Mammals carry three *RAF* genes, *A-RAF*, *B-RAF* and *C-RAF*, which reside on chromosomes Xp11, 7q34 and 3p25, respectively. The Raf proteins are structurally related and share three conserved regions (CR1, CR2 and CR3) (Figure 7). The N-terminally located CR1 contains the Ras-binding domain as well as a cysteine-rich domain, which also functions to bind Ras (185). The C-terminally located CR3 region contains the kinase domain (Figure 7).

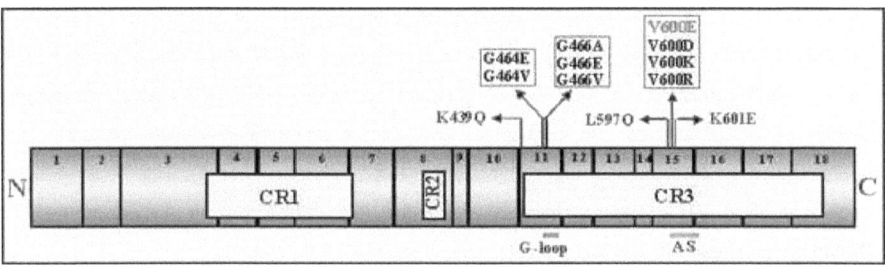

Figure 7. Diagram with B-RAF mutations found in melanoma. The black arrows indicate the mutations. Mutations inside a box are in the same amino acid. The hotspot mutation V600E is marked in red. Numbers inside the blue boxes indicate the exon from which is translated each part of the protein. The three boxes inside represent the conserved regions of the protein with the *A-RAF* and *C-RAF* genes (CR1, CR2 and CR3). A conserved glycine motif (G-loop) in exon 11 is indicated with a red bar and the activation segment (AS) in exon 15 with a pink bar. C: Carboxyl-terminal; N: Amino-terminal.

All three RAF proteins activate MEK, but with different intensities and the phenotypic differences between *A-RAF-*, *B-RAF-* and *C-RAF-*null mice suggest that the individual family members perform distinct functions in development, possibly due to differences in expression patterns (186). Neither b-raf-null nor c-raf-null mice are viable, whereas a-raf-null mice die soon after birth (187-189). B-raf-null mice die of vascular and neuronal defects (187). Whereas C-Raf is ubiquitously expressed, A-Raf and B-Raf display a more restricted expression pattern (190). Inactive cytoplasmic Raf upon binding to Ras-GTP is recruited to the cell membrane and is activated through a number of phosphorylation events.

The *B-RAF* oncogene encodes a serine/threonine kinase regulated by binding to RAS protein. B-RAF acts in the RAS/RAF/MEK/ERK pathway by transducing regulatory signals from RAS to

MEK1/2. B-RAF has a substantially greater basal kinase activity than C-RAF or A-RAF (186, 191). In contrast to C-RAF or A-RAF, B-RAF possesses only two instead of four distinct RAS-GTP-dependend phosphorylation sites for maximal activation (T599 and S602) (186, 191). This structure expedites the activation of B-RAF through a single amino acid substitution. B-RAF is expressed mainly in different neuronal tissues, but also in other cell types such as testis and heart (192).

In 2002, a genome-wide screen for proto-oncogenes showed that the *B-RAF* gene is mutated in a variety of different human cancers (193). The highest frequencies of *B-RAF* mutations were identified in melanomas (67%), colorectal (18%) and ovarian (14%) cancers (193). Over 40 different *B-RAF* mutations have been described in the literature; approximately half of those have been functionally analysed (193-195). The majority of the *B-RAF* mutations result in increased *in vitro* kinase activities of the protein; but also mutants with impaired or no kinase activity have been identified (193, 195, 196). The most common mutation found in *B-RAF* is a valine to glutamic acid change at residue 600. The V600E *B-RAF* missense mutation results in maximal constitutive activation of kinase activity. The mechanism involves a conformational change mimicking the phosphorylation at T599/S602 residues in wild-type *B-RAF* (Figure 7) (193). The V600E mutant possesses an up to 480-fold greater basal activity and induces transformation of cultured NIH3T3 cells with much higher efficiency compared to the wild-type (193, 195).

B-RAF is mutated in about 70% of melanomas (193, 197-199). Over 20 other *B-RAF* mutations described in melanoma are rather rare. *B-RAF* mutations are also found in up to 80% of melanocytic nevi, indicating that these mutations occur early during melanoma development. However, at the same time activation of B-RAF alone is insufficient to induce melanoma tumourigenesis (200-202). Spitz nevi, with histological similarity to melanoma lack *B-RAF* mutations (201, 203). Also blue nevi with characteristic colouration do not carry *B-RAF* mutations (201, 203). Expression of the V600E mutant B-raf in zebrafish results in nevi but not in melanoma formation. Expression of V600E mutant B-raf in p53-deficient fish resulted readily in invasive melanoma (204). V600E B-Raf has been shown to transform immortalised mouse melanocytes (205). Moreover, suppression of V600E B-Raf in melanoma cell lines by small interfering RNA (siRNA) resulted in less efficient growth in nude mice compared to control cells (206, 207). Melanoma cells expressing V600E *B-RAF* showed constitutive cyclin D1 expression and downregulation of the tumour suppressor p27^{Kip1} (208). Other effects reported of increased ERK activity mediated by activated B-RAF included altered integrin expression, decreased E-cadherin expression, increased MMP secretion, invasion, and the regulation of the critical melanocyte transcription factor MITF (174, 209). In contrast to cutaneous melanoma, development of uveal melanoma also seems to occur via activation of the RAS-RAF-MEK-ERK pathway, but without involvement of mutations in the *B-RAF* or *RAS* genes (210, 211).

In thyroid cancer, activation of the RAF-MEK-ERK pathway through chromosomal re-arrangement resulting in an in-frame fusion between *B-RAF* and *AKAP9* has been observed. The fusion protein, which contains the protein kinase domain and lacks the autoinhibitory N-terminal portion of B-RAF, has elevated kinase activity and transforms NIH3T3 cells. The AKAP9 – B-RAF fusion was found in radiation-induced papillary carcinomas developing after a short latency and in absence of *B-RAF* point mutations (212).

The RAS genes

The human *RAS* proto-oncogenes (*H-RAS, K-RAS,* and *N-RAS*) reside on chromosomes 11p15, 1p22 and 12p12, respectively. The three *RAS* genes encode four highly related cell membrane-associated proteins, H-Ras, N-Ras, K-Ras4A and K-Ras4B, that are involved in transduction of extracellular growth and differentiation signals (213). The four Ras proteins carry identical initial 85 amino acids. This part includes the effector domain (residues 32-40), through which Ras proteins interact with downstream effectors. The N-terminal part also contains two mobile regions named switch I (redidues 30-40) and switch II (residues 60-76) regions, both of which undergo conformational changes upon GTP binding. The most C-terminal part of Ras contains a CAAX motif. This motif is subjected to a number of post-translational modifications, which are required for the proper anchoring of Ras to the cell membrane (214).

The *RAS* genes are mutated in approximately 30% of all human tumours (215). Mutations in *K-RAS* are most common, followed by *N-RAS*, whereas mutations in *H-RAS* are rare. High frequencies of *K-RAS* alterations have been found in carcinomas of the pancreas, colon, and lung, whereas *N-RAS* mutations are frequent in myeloid leukemias and in melanomas (215). Most mutations in *RAS* genes are single base changes affecting codons 12, 13, and 61. Mutations in these codons reduce the intrinsic GTPase activity of the RAS proteins and also make them insensitive to GTPase-activating proteins (216, 217). As a result, mutated RAS is locked in the GTP-bound state and continuously activates its downstream effector targets.

The most frequent *N-RAS* mutations in melanoma occur in codon 61 (218). Mutations in codon 12 and 13 of the *N-RAS* gene are less common. The presence of *N-RAS* mutations in tumour associated nevi and RGP lesions suggests that N-RAS activation occurs at an early stage in during melanoma development (218, 219). *N-RAS* mutations are also found in 10% of common aquired nevi and 28-56% of congenital nevi (200, 202, 220). *N-RAS* mutations are associated with melanoma arising in chronically sun-exposed rather than intermittently exposed skin (221-223). Moreover, *N-RAS* mutations are rare in melanomas from sun-protected skin, indicating that UV radiation may play a role in the genesis of *N-RAS* mutations in melanoma (223). Suppression of oncogenic *N-RAS* (Q61K) in melanoma cells resulted in increased apoptosis, decreased ERK phosphorylation, and reduced expression of cyclin D1 (224). These data suggest that oncogenic *N-RAS* is important for the avoidance of apoptosis in melanoma, and imply a role of activating *N-RAS* mutations in melanoma development. Both functional and genetic evidences indicate that B-RAF and N-RAS act linearly in the RAS-RAF-MEK-ERK signalling pathway, which is evidenced by almost mutual exclusiveness of mutations in these genes and consequent ERK activation (173, 174).

Interaction between the RAS-RAF-MEK-ERK and Rb/p53 pathways
The results of several studies suggest that activated N-RAS or B-RAF alone is not able to transform human melanocytes, but require additional, cooperating events for tumour formation. Activating *B-RAF* or *N-RAS* mutations and loss of p16 expression both occur at high frequencies in melanomas. In a recent study, both the V600E mutation of *B-RAF* and p16 inactivation have been found to accompany amplification of the major melanocyte differentiation factor MITF in melanoma cell lines. MITF amplification was more prevalent in metastatic disease and correlated with decreased patient survival (225). These data identify *MITF* as a possible novel oncogene, which in cooperation with mutated B-RAF, can transform human melanocytes in a p16-deficient background. In human nevi, sustained V600E *B-RAF* expression induced cell cycle arrest, accompanied by both induction of p16 and senescence-associated acidic ß-galactosidase (SA-ß-GAL), a classical marker for senescence (42). Transgenic mice overexpressing oncogenic *N-RAS* (Q61K) did not develop melanoma, but exhibited hyper-pigmentation, and persistence of melanocytes in dermis and epidermis. Interestingly, when the *N-RAS* Q61K transgenic mice were crossed with *p19*-null knockout mice, offspring developed cutaneous metastasising melanomas within six months of birth (226). Zebrafish expressing V600E *B-RAF* develop nevi, which require a p53-deficient background to progress to invasive melanomas (204). Altogether, the results of these studies support the hypothesis, that activated N-RAS or B-RAF requires cooperating events such as p16 inactivation for melanomagenesis. Moreover, these findings underscore the importance of interaction of RAS-RAF-MEK-ERK and Rb/p53 pathways in melanoma.

1.3. GLOBAL GENE EXPRESSION ANALYSIS USING MICROARRAY TECHNOLOGY

1.3.1. Microarray technology and human cancers

Global gene expression profiles can provide comprehensive molecular portraits of biologic diversity and complex disease states. The development of microarray technology allows the simultaneous measurement of the expression of many thousands of genes in one single experiment while previous methods have only allowed measurements of single genes. By enabling studies on a genome-wide scale, microarray technology is currently revolutionising biological research and creating a wide range of research opportunities. This high-throughput technique can be used to predict the function of unknown genes, in medical diagnostics, in biomarker discovery, to infer networks from the regulatory interactions between genes, and to investigate the mechanisms by which a drug, disease, mutation and environmental condition affects gene expression and cell function. Global gene expression profiles have the potential to better define biologic phenomena and human disease states at the molecular level. A particular application of the microarray technology is in cancer research, where the goal is a precise and early diagnosis of tumorous malignancies, allowing for a tailored treatment with less side-effects and higher cure rates. Based on the differential expression of hundreds to thousands of genes, many cancers previously thought to be homogenuous are now recognised to consist of distinct molecular subtypes and are often associated with significantly different clinical outcomes (227, 228). In breast cancer studies, gene expression profiling has been used to improve the prognostication for primary breast cancer patients, and has had particular success in reducing the requirement for adjuvant therapy (229, 230). Microarray analyses have also been applied to several dermatologic diseases, including melanoma, psoriasis, and scleroderma (231-233).

1.3.2. Gene expression profiling of malignant melanoma

Elucidating the fundamental molecular mechanisms that are involved in the stepwise progression from normal tissues to malignant tumours is essential in the knowledge of cancers. Melanoma is ideal for the study of mechanisms involved in the stepwise progression of the disease from normal pigment cells to atypical nevi to invasive primary melanoma and finally to cells with aggressive metastatic potential. With a series of mutational events, normal melanocytes are transformed into dysplastic cells that then progress to invasive melanoma cells capable of metastatic spread throughout the body. It is presumed that multiple genetic alterations lead to complex patterns of gene expression resulting in transformation and progression of the disease (234). Microarray technology allows to study the regulation of gene expression in the sequence of steps that take place from the normal melanocytic cell to malignant melanoma and to identify novel disease-related genes more rapidly and with greater accuracy. Different microarray studies using melanoma cell lines or primary tumours identified numerous genes associated with melanoma progression (231, 235-238). Such genes include *MCP-1, TRP-1, WAF-1, RhoC, WNT5A*, fibronectin, integrins β1 and β3, *BCL-2,* and *MMP-14.* (231, 235, 236, 239, 240). Recently, microarray-based gene expression signatures of different *B-RAF* and *N-RAS* mutations have been identified (241). With regard to malignant melanoma, microarray technology is a promising application to identify global gene expression alterations that are involved in the different stages of disease development. These line of investigation contributes to the improvement of screening methods to identify individuals at increased risk of developing melanoma and to the design of treatments using gene-directed therapy.

2. AIMS OF THE STUDY

The general aim of this thesis was to characterize somatic alterations in specific cancer-related genes and their effects on global gene expression in cutaneous malignant melanoma. Those genes include the *B-RAF* and *N-RAS* proto-oncogenes, as well as the *CDKN2A* tumour suppressor gene. The studies were performed on a large series of melanoma cell lines and melanocytic nevi.

Specific aims were:

1. To evaluate the frequency of mutations in *B-RAF* and *N-RAS* genes and alterations of the *CDKN2A* gene in melanoma cell lines
2. To determine the level of expression of B-RAF, N-RAS and CDKN2A in melanoma cell lines
    (a) To determine the frequency of the AKAP9 – B-RAF fusion transcript in melanoma cell lines
3. To evaluate
    (a) the effect of common *B-RAF* and *N-RAS* mutations on global gene expression in melanoma cell lines
    (b) differences in global gene expression in melanoma cell lines with and without homozygous deletions of the *CDKN2A* locus genes
    (c) the effect of the common V600E *B-RAF* mutation on global gene expression in melanocytic nevi

3. MATERIALS AND METHODS

3.1. MELANOMA CELL LINES

3.1.1. Cell lines and cell culture

A panel of 140 melanoma cell lines derived from 106 individual patients were included in the present studies. The patients were followed up at the Department of Dermatology, University Hospital Mannheim. Melanoma cell lines were established from solid metastatic lesions or malignant effusions. Patient´s characteristics were available for 85 of the 106 patients (Table 2).

Table 2. Characteristics of melanoma cell lines and patients.

		Cell lines 85 (100.0%)
Gender	male	44 (52)
	female	41 (48)
Age[*]	(median/range)	56 (age 17-87)
Stage (AJCC)[*]	III	17 (20)
	IV	68 (80)
Location of primary tumour	skin	66 (78)
	mucosa	1 (1)
	occult	11 (13)
	n.a.	27 (32)
Type of primary tumour	NM	24 (28)
	SSM	17 (20)
	ALM	5 (6)
	LMM	1 (1)
	occult	11 (13)
	n.a.	27 (32)
Origin of cells for mutation analysis	skin/subcutis met	41 (48)
	lymph node met	33 (40)
	organ met	4 (5)
	malignant effusion	7 (8)

* the patient´s age and disease stage refer to the time point of cell extraction. n.a., not available; met, metastasis

Cell lines were established by mincing the tumour specimens and maintained in RPMI 1640 supplemented with 10% fetal calf serum (both from Life Technologies, Grand Island, NY, USA), 5 mM L-glutamine, 100 U/ml penicillin and 100 µg/ml streptomycin at 37°C in a humidified 5%

carbon dioxide (CO_2) atmosphere. Cell lines were used for analysis no latter than six to eight passages. For isolation of DNA/RNA all cell lines were cultured until 70-80% confluence, gently detached by 0.05% ethylenediaminetetra-acetic (EDTA)/phosphate buffered-saline (PBS), washed twice, re-suspended in 10% fetal calf serum/RPMI and frozen down in liquid nitrogen until further analysis.

3.1.2. Isolation of DNA and RNA

2×10^6 cells were used from each cell line to isolate genomic DNA and total RNA using commercially available purification kits (Purescript/Puregene, Gentra Systems, Minneapolis, MN). 300 µl cell lysis solution were added to the cell pellet. Proteins and DNA were precipitated by adding 100 µl protein-DNA precipitation solution to the cell lysate. The cell lysate was inverted 10 times and placed on ice for 5 minutes. A pellet of precipitated proteins and DNA was obtained by centrifugation at 13 000 rpm for 10 minutes at 4°C. The pellet was stored for subsequent DNA isolation. Total RNA was precipitated from the supernatant with 300 µl 100% ice-cold isopropanol and centrifuged at 13 000 rpm for 5 minutes at 4°C. RNA was washed with 300 µl 70% ethanol and a final centrifugation was carried out at 13 000 rpm for 5 minutes. RNA was air-dried for 15 minutes and then resuspended in 50 µl RNA hydration solution. Total RNA was subjected to a second cleanup by a silica-gel-based membrane using RNeasy Mini Kit (Qiagen, Hilden, Germany).

DNA was isolated from DNA-protein precipitate by resuspending in 300 µl cell lysis solution. The cell lysate was incubated at 37°C until the solution was homogenuous. Residual RNA was degraded by incubating the cell lysate with 1.5 µl RNase A solution at 37°C for 15 minutes. Proteins were precipitated by adding 100 µl protein precipitation solution to the cell lysate and vortexing at high speed for 20 seconds. The cell solution was centrifuged at 13 000 rpm for 5 minutes. DNA was precipitated from the supernatant with 300 µl 100% isopropanol and centrifuged at 13 000 rpm for 5 minutes. DNA was washed with 300 µl 70% ethanol and a final centrifugation was carried out at 13 000 rpm for 5 minutes. The DNA pellet was air-dried for 15 minutes and then resuspended in 50 µl DNA hydration solution. Concentrations of DNA and RNA were measured by UV spectrophotometry and OD 260/280 nm ratios between 1.9 and 2.1 were obtained for all DNA and RNA samples. The integrity of RNA isolated from cell lines was determined on Bioanalyzer 2100 System (Agilent Technologies, Palo Alto, CA) using 400 ng RNA from each cell line.

3.1.3. DNA sequencing

DNA isolated from all melanoma cell lines was screened for mutations in exons 11 and 15 of the *B-RAF* gene, exons 1 and 2 of the *N-RAS* gene and exons 1α, 1β, 2 and 3 of the *CDKN2A* gene using gene-specific primers given in Table 3 and described earlier (126, 197).

Table 3. Primers used for PCR amplification of exons in different genes.

Gene	Primer	Sequence	Fragment length
B-RAF			
Exon 11	BrafEx11F	5´-CTC TCA GGC ATA AGG TAA TG-3´	
	BrafEx11R2	5´-TTG ATG CGA ACA GTG AAT-3´	316 bp
Exon 15	BrafEx15F	5´-CCT AAA CTC TTC ATA ATG CTT-3´	
	BrafEx15R	5´-ATA GCC TCA ATT CTT ACC AT-3´	209 bp
N-RAS			
Exon 1	NrasEx1F	5´-CGC AAA TTA ACC CTG ATT ACT-3´	
	NrasEx1R	5´-CAC TGG GCC TCA CCT CTA-3´	174 bp
Exon 2	NrasEx2F	5´-CCC CCA CGA TTC TTA CAG A-3´	
	NrasEx2R	5´-AGG TTA ATA TCC GCA AAT GAC-3´	180 bp
CDKN2A			
Exon 1α	CDKN2AEx1aF	5´-CGG CTG CGG AGA GGG GGA GAG-3´	
	CDKN2AEx1aR	5´-CTC CAG AGT CGC CCG CCA TCC-3´	246 bp
Exon 1β	CDKN2AEx1bF	5´-GGA GGC GGC GAG AAC AT-3´	
	CDKN2AEx1bR	5´-GGG CCT TTC CTA CCT GGT CTT-3´	221 bp
Exon 2	CDKN2AEx2-5endF	5´-GGG CTC TAC ACA AGC TTC CTT-3´	
	CDKN2AEx2-3endR	5´-TTT GGA AGC TCT CAG GGT ACA-3´	425 bp
Exon 3	CDKN2AEx3F	5´-GCC TGT TTT CTT TCT GCC CTC TG-3´	
	CDKN2AEx3R	5´-CGA AAG CGG GGT GGG TTG T-3´	143 bp

PCR amplification

Exons 11 and 15 of *B-RAF* and exons 1 and 2 of *N-RAS* were amplified in a 13-µl volume reaction. Each reaction contained 10 ng DNA, 1 x PCR buffer, 1.5 mM magnesium chloride, 0.11 mM of each dNTP (Invitrogen, Paisley, UK), 0.3 µM forward and reverse primer, respectively (MWG Biotech AG, Ebersberg, Germany), 0.3 U Platinum Taq Polymerase (Invitrogen) and dH$_2$O. PCR was carried out in a GeneAmp 9700 PCR System (Applied Biosystems, Foster City, USA). Initial denaturation was performed at 94°C for 1 minute, followed by 3 cycles each consisting of denaturation at 94°C for 45 seconds, annealing at 60°C for 45 seconds and extension at 72°C for 45 seconds. Additional 32 cycles were performed each consisting of denaturation at 94°C for 30 seconds, annealing at 59°C for 30 seconds and extension at 72°C for 30 seconds, followed by a final extension at 72°C for 5 minutes. Two µl of the PCR product were subsequently analysed on a 1%

agarose gel (Sigma, Munich, Germany), stained by ethidium bromide, which was run at a constant voltage of 120V in 1 x TAE (40 mM Tris acetate, 1 mM EDTA) for 30 minutes.

Sequencing reaction

In order to remove residual primers and nucleotides, PCR products were incubated with ExoSapIT (USB Amersham, Uppsala, Sweden) at 37°C for 30 minutes, followed by heating to 85°C for 15 minutes. The sequencing reactions were carried out using the BigDye Terminator Cycle Sequencing Kit (Applied Biosystems). The primers used for sequencing were those used for PCR amplification of the DNA (Table 3). The sequencing reaction was performed in a 10-µl set up containing 1 µl purified PCR product, 10 µM sequencing primer, 1.75 µl of sequencing buffer, 0.5 µl of BigDye Premix and dH_2O. The temperature conditions were 94°C for 10 seconds followed by 28 cycles at 94°C for 10 seconds, 55°C for 5 seconds and 60°C for 3 minutes. Final extension was performed at 60°C for 1 second. The reaction products were precipitated using final concentrations of 80 mM sodium acetate, pH 4.6 and 70% ethanol. After vortexing the precipitation mix was centrifuged at 4000 rpm for 45 minutes. The supernatant was removed and the DNA was washed with 70% ethanol. After a second centrifugation step at 4000 rpm for 15 minutes and removal of the supernatant, DNA was air-dried and resuspended in 20 µl dH_2O. The DNA was analysed on an ABI Prism 3100 Genetic Analyzer (Applied Biosystems). Forward and reverse strands were sequenced separately. Primary sequencing data were analysed using a sequence analysis software (Sequence Analysis 3.7; Applied Biosystems). Comparative analysis was done using the MultAlin algorithm (http://www.prodes.toulouse.inra.fr/multalin/multalin.html) and DNAStar software.

3.1.4. Global gene expression in melanoma cells

Cell lines used for microarray analysis
Three cell lines with V600E mutation in the *B-RAF* gene; four cell lines with Q61R mutation in the *N-RAS* gene; four melanoma cell lines (derived from three individual patients) with homozygous deletion of the *CDKN2A* locus; and three cell lines without mutations in the *B-RAF* and *N-RAS* genes or homozygous deletion at the *CDKN2A* locus were selected for the microarray expression experiments. Cell lines chosen for this investigation were established from tissue specimens of metastasised lesions from cutaneous melanoma (Table 4).

Sample preparation, hybridisation, washing and scanning
An overview of the eukaryotic sample and array processing is given in Figure 8. Total RNA isolated from tissues or cells is reverse transcribed into double-stranded complementary DNA (cDNA). An *in vitro* transcription (IVT) reaction is then performed to produce biotin-labeled amplified RNA (aRNA) from the cDNA. Before hybridisation the aRNA is fragmented.

Table 4. Melanoma cell lines used for gene expression analysis.

Mutation	Cell line code	Origin
without mutation	UKRV-Mel-4	liver metastases
	UKRV-Mel-5	cutaneous/sub-cutaneous lesion
	UKRV-Mel-11	lymph node metastases
B-RAF V600E	Ma-Mel-16a	small bowel metastases
	Ma-Mel-51	lymph node metastases
	Ma-Mel-57	lymph node metastases
N-RAS Q61R	UKRV-Mel-15d	lymph node metastases
	UKRV-Mel-19a	lymph node metastases
	Ma-Mel-28	cutaneous/sub-cutaneous lesion
	Ma-Mel-43	cutaneous/sub-cutaneous lesion
CDKN2A homozygous deletion	Ma-Mel-2	cutaneous/sub-cutaneous lesion
	Ma-Mel-8a	cutaneous/sub-cutaneous lesion
	Ma-Mel-8b	cutaneous/sub-cutaneous lesion
	Ma-Mel-40	cutaneous/sub-cutaneous lesion

During hybridisation, the biotin-labeled aRNA binds to complementary oligonucleotide probes attached on the microarray. The hybridised probe array is stained with streptavidin phycoerythrin conjugate and scanned at an excitation wavelength of 488 nm. The amount of light emitted at 570 nm is proportional to the bound target at each location on the microarray.

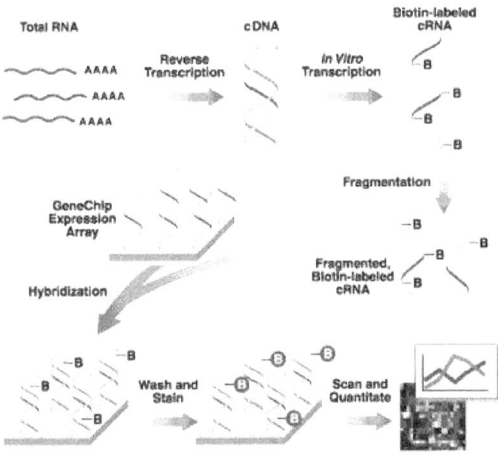

Figure 8. Overview of sample processing of the eukaryotic gene expression assay. [source: http://cnx.rice.edu/content/m12388/latest/]

Two µg of total RNA from each cell line was converted into double-stranded cDNA using SuperScript Double-Stranded cDNA Synthesis Kit (Invitrogen, Carlsbad, CA). First strand synthesis was carried out using 50 µM T7-oligo(dT) primer (QIAGEN, Hilden, Germany) as per the manufacturer's instructions. Second strand synthesis was performed at 16°C for 2 hours in a final volume of 150 µl as per the manufacturer's recommendations. The double-stranded cDNA was cleaned up with the GeneChip Sample Cleanup Module (Affymetrix, Sunnydale, CA).

12 µl of the purified cDNA were used for synthesis of biotin-labeled aRNA using ENZO Labeling Kit (Enzo, Farmingdale, NY). In vitro transcription (IVT) reaction in a total volume of 40 µl was set up as per the manufacturer's instructions and incubated at 37°C for 16 hours. 20 µg cleaned-up biotin-labeled aRNA from each reaction was cut into 35-200 bp fragments in a 40 µl volume reaction containing 8 µl 5 x fragmentation buffer (Affymetrix, Sunnydale, CA) and dH$_2$O. Fragmentation was carried out at 94°C for 35 minutes. Gel electrophoresis was performed to verify the expected size distribution of unfragmented and fragmented aRNA.

5 µg of fragmented aRNA from each cell line was hybridised on Affymetrix Test3 arrays in order to test the entire procedure. Only those aRNA samples that showed at least 27% present calls and 3´ to 5´ signal ratios of 0.9 - 1.5 for the housekeeping genes ß-actin (*ACTB*) and glyceinaldehyd-3-phosphat-dehydrogenase (*GAPDH*) on the test arrays were loaded on Human Genome HG-

U133A2.0 microarrays (Affymetrix, Inc.) with 22 277 probe sets corresponding to 14 500 genes. 10 µg of fragmented labeled aRNA was hybridized onto the array at 45°C for 16 hours. A 200 µl hybridisation cocktail included 50 pM control oligonucleotide B2, 1.5, 5, 25 and 100 pM, respectively, as eukaryotic hybridisation controls, 0.1 mg/ml herring sperm DNA, 0.5 mg/ml acetylated bovine serum albumin (BSA), 1 x hybridisation buffer and dH$_2$O. Before loading on the arrays, the hybridization cocktails were denaturated at 99°C for 5 minutes, transferred to 45°C, incubated for 5 minutes and then centrifuged for 5 minutes at 14 000 rpm to pellet debris. After hybridisation, washing and staining was carried out using a fluidics station (GeneChip Fluidics Station 400, Affymetrix) and a confocal scanner, according to the manufacturer's instructions (Affymetrix). In brief, the hybridised probe array was washed and stained with a streptavidin phycoerythrin conjugate (Invitrogen, Paisley, UK) followed by a signal amplification step and performed using biotinylated anti-streptavidin antibody (Vector Laboratories, Burlingame, USA). The arrays were scanned by the GeneChip Scanner 3100 at the excitation wavelength of 488 nm. The amount of light emitted at 570 nm is proportional to the bound target at each location on the microarray.

3.2. MELANOCYTIC NEVI

3.2.1. Origin /Subjects

The study included thirty benign melanocytic nevi obtained from ten individuals. The individuals were recruited from the Päijät-Häme Central Hospital (Prof. Erna Snellman), Lahti, Finland. The sampling was carried out in accordance with the Helsinki Declaration. All subjects were healthy individuals, with no history of melanoma or any other skin cancers (Table 5).

Table 5. Types of benign melanocytic nevi and mutations detected in the *B-RAF* and *N-RAS* genes. Nevi used for expression analysis are underlined and marked in bold.

Individual No.	Nevus No.	Mutation	Site	Gender/Age of Person	Nevus count	Skin cancer in family
1	**1**	**V600E *B-RAF***	abdomen	M/42	2-10	no
	2	**V600E *B-RAF***	breast/side			
2	**3**	**V600E *B-RAF***	upper back	F/39	11-50	Cousin and uncle had melanoma
	4	**V600E *B-RAF***	upper back			
	5	**V600E *B-RAF***	upper back			
3	**6**	**V600E *B-RAF***	mid-back	M/23	51-100	no
	7	**V600E *B-RAF***	breast/side			
	8	**V600E *B-RAF***	shoulder			
4	**9**	**None**	shoulder	F/35	51-100	no
	10	None	abdomen			
5	11	V600E *B-RAF*	back	F/40	>100	no
	12	**None**	side			
	13	**None**	side			
6	14	V600E *B-RAF*	back, scapula	M/38	11-50	Uncle had melanoma
	15	**V600E *B-RAF***	abdomen			
	16	**V600E *B-RAF***	abdomen			
7	17	Q61K *N-RAS*	thigh	F/33	>100	Mother and grandmother had melanoma
	18	Q61R *N-RAS*	shoulder			
	19	**V600E *B-RAF***	shoulder			
	20	**V600E *B-RAF***	shoulder			
	21	V600E *B-RAF*	shoulder			
8	**22**	**V600E *B-RAF***	abdomen	M/42	51-100	no
	23	**V600E *B-RAF***	abdomen			
	24	**V600E *B-RAF***	abdomen			
9	25	V600E *B-RAF*	neck	F/27	51-100	no
	26	**V600E *B-RAF***	back			
	27	**V600E *B-RAF***	back			
	28	**V600E *B-RAF***	thigh			
10	**29**	**None**	abdomen	F/47	51-100	no
	30	V600E *B-RAF*	abdomen			

The mean age of the individuals was 43.0 (± 17.0) years. The nevus tissue was taken by punch biopsy from the middle of the moles. The rest, including residual nevus and non-nevus tissues, were excised in boat-shaped cuts. The moles were assessed for colour, border, and symmetry and only symmetrical, benign-looking moles with no recent change in outlook were removed for the study. The clinical type of the mole (junctional, compound, or intradermal) and their colour were defined before biopsy. In this study nine non-nevus tissue samples were included, provided by the Department of Dermatology, University Hospital Mannheim (Prof. Dirk Schadendorf).

3.2.2. Isolation of DNA and RNA

For isolation of DNA and RNA each nevus tissue after excision of fat was cut into two. One part was used for isolation of DNA and the second for isolation of RNA. Total RNA was isolated from nevus tissue using a commercially available kit (RNeasy Micro Kit, Qiagen, Hilden, Germany). Nevus tissue was homogenised using a Tissuelyser (Qiagen, Hilden, Germany). Tissue disruption was achieved through the beating and grinding effect of stainless steel beads (5 mm diameter), which were shaken with the tissue in the grinding vessel. Nevus tissue, together with 150 µl cell lysis buffer and one bead was shaken 2 x 1 minute at a frequency of 30 Hertz. 295 µl dH$_2$O and 5 µl proteinase K were added to the homogenate followed by incubation for 10 minutes at 55°C. After centrifugation at 12 000 rpm for 3 minutes at room temperature, precipitation was carried out by adding of 0.5 volumes of 100% ethanol to the supernatant. The sample was applied to a spin column and centrifuged for 15 seconds at 10 000 rpm.

A wash step was carried out using 350 µl wash buffer and centrifugation for 15 seconds at 10 000 rpm. DNA was digested by incubation with 27 U of DNase I on the column at room temperature for 15 minutes. After incubation, 350 µl wash buffer was pipetted onto the column followed by centrifugation for 15 seconds at 10 000 rpm. The wash step was repeated with 500 µl wash buffer containing ethanol and centrifugation at 15 seconds at 10 000 rpm. A third wash step was performed with 500 µl 80% ethanol and centrifugation at 10 000 rpm for 2 minutes. The column was dried by final centrifugation at 13 000 rpm for 5 minutes. RNA was eluted after incubation with 14 µl dH$_2$O for 3 minutes at room temperature and centrifugation at 13 000 rpm for 1 minute. Concentration of RNA was measured with an UV-Vis Spectrophotometer (NanoDrop Technologies, Wilmington, USA) and OD 260/280 nm ratios between 1.8 and 2.0 were obtained for all RNA samples. The integrity of total RNA isolated from melanocytic nevi was determined on Bioanalyzer 2100 System (Agilent Technologies, Palo Alto, CA) using 5 ng RNA isolated from each nevus.

For isolation of genomic DNA, homogenisation of nevus tissue was carried out as described above. After RNase and proteinase K digestion DNA was isolated by phenol-chloroform extraction in our laboratory by other colleagues (A. Gast and R. Thirumaran).

3.2.3. Mutation detection

DNA from thirty melanocytic nevi was screened for mutations in exons 11 and 15 of the *B-RAF* gene and exons 1 and 2 of the *N-RAS* gene with radioactive single strand conformation polymorphism (SSCP) technique by other colleagues (S. Angelini, A. Gast and R. Thirumaran).

3.2.4. Global gene expression in melanocytic nevi

Melanocytic nevi used for microarray analysis
Total RNA from eighteen nevi with V600E *B-RAF* mutation was chosen for the microarray experiments. Of the seven nevi with no mutation in *B-RAF* or *N-RAS*, RNA was available from only four nevi for this study (Table 5). Nine non-nevus tissue samples were also included in the study.

Sample preparation, hybridisation, washing and scanning
Samples for microarray analysis were prepared using the BioArray RNA Amplification and Labeling System (Enzo, Farmingdale, NY). Biotin-labeled amplified RNA was obtained in a two-round amplification procedure of 100 ng total RNA according to the manufacturer's protocol (Figure 9).

• *First round of amplification*
First strand cDNA synthesis was carried out in a 20 µl volume reaction containing 100 ng total RNA, 1 µl undiluted low input T7-dT primer, 2 µl first strand buffer, 1 µl dNTP mix, 2 µl DTT solution, 1 µl reverse transcriptase mix and dH$_2$O. The reaction mix was incubated at 42°C for 1 hour. After incubation remaining RNA was degraded by adding 20 µl RNA eliminator to the reaction and incubation at 37°C for 20 minutes. The solution was then neutralised by adding 2 µl neutralizer. First strand cDNA was was purified using a commercial kit (Qiagen, Hilden, Germany) according to the modified protocol specified in the BioArray manual. A homopolymeric tail was added at the 3´end of the purified first strand cDNA. The tailing mix was prepared containing 3 µl TdT buffer, 3 µl cobaltous chloride (CoCl$_2$) solution, 1 µl tailing nucleotide, 1 µl terminal transferase and dH$_2$O up to a volume of 11 µl and added to the purified cDNA. The tailing reaction

was carried out at 37°C for 15 minutes. After tailing, chain termination was performed by adding 0.5 µl TdT buffer, 2 µl magnesium chloride solution, 1 µl terminator, 0.5 µl terminal transferase and 1 µl dH$_2$O to the tailing mix. The termination mix was incubated at 37°C for 15 minutes. Subsequently, 9 µl 5 x protease buffer and 1 µl protease were added and incubation was prolonged for further 15 minutes at 37°C. The tailed and terminated first strand cDNA was purified using a commercial kit (Qiagen, Hilden, Germany). Second strand synthesis was performed at 42°C for 1 hour in a final volume of 20 µl by adding 1 µl undiluted low input primer 2, 6 µl second strand buffer, 3 µl dNTP mix and 1 µl DNA polymerase to the first strand cDNA. Double-stranded cDNA was cleaned up as described above. The entire amount of purified double-stranded cDNA was used for synthesis of aRNA.

In vitro transcription (IVT) reaction in a total volume of 40 µl that contained 19 µl cDNA, 4 µl 10 x IVT reaction buffer, 4 µl ribonucleotide mix (unlabeled), 4 µl 10 x DTT solution, 4 µl 10 x RNase inhibitor mix, 2 µl 20 x T7 RNA polymerase and 3 µl dH$_2$O was incubated at 37°C for 16 hours. Amplified RNA was purified with a commercially available kit (Qiagen, Hilden, Germany) according to the modified protocol in the BioArray manual. 1 µl of aRNA was used for quantification by an UV-Vis Spectrophotometer (NanoDrop Technologies, Wilmington, USA). Amplified RNA yields after the first round of amplification ranged from 400 – 800 ng.

For the second round of amplification samples were concentrated by precipitation to a final volume of 12 µl. Therefore, 10 µg glycogen (Invitrogen, Paisley, UK), 0.5 volumes 5M ammonium acetate (Ambion, Huntingdon, UK) and 2.5 volumes 100% ethanol were added to the eluted aRNA and the mixture was incubated at -20°C for 30 minutes. Subsequently, the solution was centrifuged at 13 000 rpm for 15 minutes at room temperature and the supernatant was removed. The pellet was washed with ice-cold 70% ethanol followed by centrifugation at 13 000 rpm for 10 minutes at room temperature. After removal of the supernatant the RNA was air-dried for 10 minutes and then resuspended in 12 µl of nuclease-free H$_2$O.

▪ *Second round of amplification*
First and second strand cDNA synthesis were carried out with undiluted high input primer using the reagents and conditions described for the first and second strand synthesis in the first round of amplification. Instead of the low input T7-dT primer, now 1 µl of was used for each reaction. Complementary DNA was purified using a commercial kit (Qiagen, Hilden, Germany) according to

the modified protocol specified in the BioArray manual. The entire amount of purified double-stranded cDNA was used for synthesis of aRNA.

In vitro transcription (IVT) reaction was carried out with biotin-labeled ribonucleotides using reagents and conditions described for the first round of amplification. Biotin-labeled amplified RNA was purified as described above. 1 µl of aRNA was used for quantification by an UV-Vis Spectrophotometer (NanoDrop Technologies, Wilmington, USA). Biotin-labeled aRNA yields after the second round of amplification ranged from 30-70 µg.

▪ *Fragmentation and Hybridisation*
17 µg biotin-labeled aRNA from each reaction was cut into 35-200 bp fragments in a 40 µl volume reaction containing 8 µl 5 x fragmentation buffer (Affymetrix, Sunnydale, CA) and dH$_2$O at 94°C for 35 minutes. 5 µg of fragmented aRNA from each nevus was hybridised on Affymetrix Test3 arrays in order to test the entire amplification procedure. Subsequently, 10 µg of fragmented aRNA were hybridised onto Human Genome HG-U133A2.0 microarrays (Affymetrix, Inc.) at 45°C for 16 hours. A 200 µl hybridisation cocktail included 50 pM control oligonucleotide B2, 1.5, 5, 25 and 100 pM, respectively, as eukaryotic hybridisation controls, 0.1 mg/ml herring sperm DNA, 0.5 mg/ml acetylated bovine serum albumin (BSA), 1 x hybridisation buffer and dH$_2$O. After hybridisation the microarrays were stained, washed and scanned as described under 3.1.4..

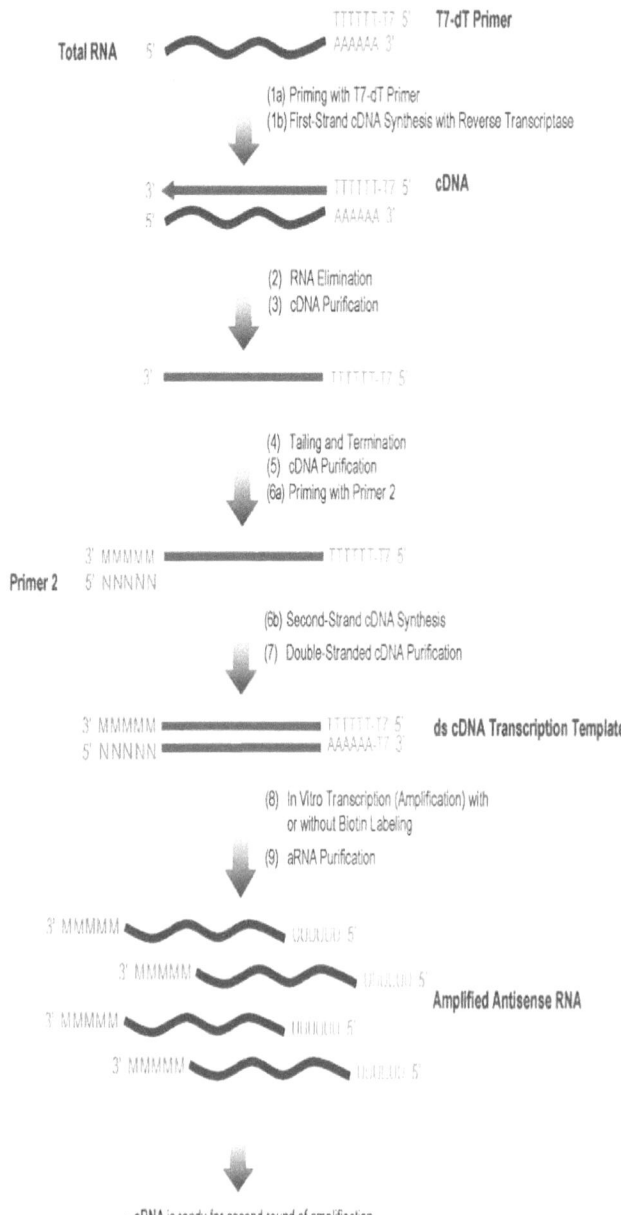

Figure 9. Overview of the two-round amplification procedure using BioArray RNA Amplification and Labeling System. [source: ENZO Bioarray RNA Amplification and Labeling System Manual]

3.3. MICROARRAY DATA ANALYSIS

3.3.1. Image Analysis

Scanned output files were visually inspected for hybridisation artifacts and then analysed with the Affymetrix GeneChip Operating Software (GCOS). To allow comparison of gene expression, the arrays were globally scaled to an average intensity of 100. Image analysis was performed to convert intensities to a numerical format and to obtain a detection call. This call indicated whether a transcript was reliably detected (Present) or not detected (Absent). A detection p-value, which is calculated using the One-Sided Wilcoxon´s Signed Rank test, reflects the confidence of the detection call. Additionally, a signal value was calculated for each probe set on the array using the One-Step Tukey´s Biweight Estimate, which assigns a relative measure of abundance to the transcript. Target intensities from each array were scaled to a value of 100. The statistical algorithms used are described in further detail in Affymetrix 2002 GeneChip Expression Analysis at http://www.affymetrix.com/Download/manuals/data_analysis_fundamentals_manual.pdf.

3.3.2. GeneChip Operating Software (GCOS)

GCOS was used for pair-wise comparisons of expression profiles between melanoma cell lines with mutation in the *B-RAF* and *N-RAS* genes or homozygous deletion of the *CDKN2A* locus and cell lines without mutations or deletions, which were designated as baseline arrays. Similarly, melanocytic nevi harbouring *B-RAF* mutation were compared to those without mutation and non-nevus tissues. Furthermore, melanocytic nevi were compared with non-nevus skin tissues. During comparison analysis, each probe set on the experimental array was compared with its counterpart on the baseline array and a change in P-value was calculated indicating the change call: "increase", "marginal increase", "decrease", "marginal decrease" or "no change" in gene expression. A second algorithm was used to calculate a quantitative estimate of the gene expression change in the form of Signal Log Ratio. A Signal Log Ratio of 1 or -1 corresponded to an increase or decrease, respectively, in transcript level by 2-fold. Further analysis that included sorting of data and identification of overlaps between changed probes was done by using Data Mining Tool Software (Affymetrix). Probe sets, that were "absent" in both baseline samples and experimental samples were excluded. Secondly, comparisons with a "no change" call were removed. For identification of differentially expressed genes two criteria were applied, (a) change of expression level of ´2-fold or more´ (which equals to SLR of at least 1 or -1, respectively) and (b) 100% concordance in increase or decrease of expression in each single comparison.

3.3.3. Significance Analysis of Microarrays (SAM)

SAM identifies genes with statistically significant changes in expression by assimilating a set of gene-specific *t*-tests. Each gene is assigned a score by SAM on the basis of a change in gene expression relative to the standard deviation of repeated experiments. When a gene is scored higher than a user-selected threshold, SAM uses a permutation of the repeated experiments to estimate the percentage of genes identified by chance (the false discovery rate [FDR]). For comparison of melanoma cell lines with *B-RAF* mutation and cell lines without the mutation we chose delta=1.05 and R=2 (2-fold change or more) to obtain a number of up- and downregulated probes numerically comparable to the number of probes obtained from analysis using the two other data analysis softwares. The resulting data set yielded an estimated false discovery rate of 18.5%. Similarly, to compare *N-RAS* mutated cell lines with cell lines without mutation a delta value of 1.59 and R=2 were chosen with 7.3% FDR. For comparison of cell lines with *CDKN2A* deletions and cell lines without deletion we chose delta=1.037 and R=2 with an estimated false discovery rate of 12.9% to obtain probe lists of up- and downregulated probe sets which are numerically comparable to the probe lists obtained from the other two softwares (GCOS and GeneCluster2.0).

3.3.4. GeneCluster2.0

Marker Analysis was performed using GeneCluster2.0 to identify genes correlated with particular class distinction, cell lines and melanocytic nevi with versus without the mutation. The default settings for the filtering procedure were used as follows: genes were excluded if they exhibited <3-fold (max/min) and 100 U (max-min) absolute variations across the dataset after a threshold of 20 U and a ceiling of 16 000 U were applied. The threshold of 20 U was set to avoid missing any potentially informative marker genes. Normalisation of the dataset was performed by standardising each row (probe set) to mean=0 and variance=1. To compare neighbours in the marker analysis a class template was created. For analysis of expression data obtained from melanoma cell lines we chose 300 markers for each class for this analysis to obtain probe lists numerically similar to those obtained by GCOS and SAM softwares for purpose of comparison. We analysed cell lines with *B-RAF* mutation, *N-RAS* mutation or *CDKN2A* deletion separately and data from cell lines without mutations were used as a baseline. The gene ranking method "Signal to Noise" was selected, which identified the difference of means in each of the classes scaled by the sum of standard deviations. The "Signal to Noise" statistics assigns a lower ranking score to genes that have higher variance in each class more than those genes that have a high variance in one class and a low variance in another.

3.3.5. Identification of differentially expressed genes

For gene identification and annotation, the data were applied to the Netaffx Analysis Center (http://www.affymetrix.com), which maps the Affymetrix probe identifiers to gene identities including links to the Gene Ontology Mining Tool and Pathway Softwares.

3.4. QUANTITATIVE REAL-TIME PCR

3.4.1. Validation of microarray expression results

The expression data from the microarray experiments were validated by quantitative real-time PCR. The mRNA levels of five genes showing significant upregulation and four genes with significant downregulation in melanoma cell lines with mutations compared to the ones without mutations were assessed by quantitative real-time PCR (Table 6).

Table 6. Validation of microarray data by quantitative real-time PCR. Selected genes showing significant up- or downregulation in melanoma cell lines with mutations or deletions.

Gene name	Mutational status of melanoma cell lines
Upregulated	
dual-specificity phosphatase 6 (*DUSP6*) v-akt murine thymoma viral oncogene homolog 3 (*AKT3*)	V600E *B-RAF*, Q61R *N-RAS*, *CDKN2A* homozygous deletion
sprouty homolog 2 (*SPRY2*)	V600E *B-RAF*, *CDKN2A* homozygous deletion
transcriptional coactivator with PDZ-binding motif (*TAZ*)	V600E *B-RAF*, *CDKN2A* homozygous deletion
matrix metalloproteinase 14 (*MMP14*)	V600E *B-RAF*
Downregulated	
Interleukin 18 (*IL18*) Krüppel-like factor 5 (*KLF5*) Inhibitor of DNA binding 2 (*ID2*) Programmed cell death 4 (*PDCD4*)	V600E *B-RAF*, Q61R *N-RAS*, *CDKN2A* homozygous deletion

cDNA was synthesised using 1 µg of total RNA (from the same batch as used in micro-array experiments) from each cell line with First Strand cDNA Synthesis Kit (Fermentas Life Sciences, St. Leon-Rot, Germany). A 20 µl volume reaction contained 0.5 µg oligo(dT)$_{18}$ primer, 1 x reaction buffer, 20 U RiboLock ribonuclease inhibitor, 1 mM dNTP mix, 40 U M-MuLV reverse transcriptase and dH$_2$O. The reaction mix was incubated at 37°C for 60 minutes following heat inactivation at 70°C for 10 minutes. cDNA samples were frozen at -80°C in small single-use aliquots until used.

Real-time PCR was carried out on an ABI PRISM 7900 Sequence Detection System (Applied Biosystems, Foster City, CA) and results were analysed using the integrated Sequence Detection System Software Version 2.1. Reverse transcription reaction equivalent to 10 ng RNA was used, in triplicate, to amplify each cDNA using gene specific primers and probes. The real-time PCR was carried out in a final volume of 20 µl containing 9 µl of diluted cDNA sample, 1 x TaqMan Universal Master Mix with AmpErase UNG (uracil-N-glycosylase) and 1 x TaqMan Gene Expression Assay (Applied Biosystems, Foster City, CA). Thermocycle program was set at initial hold at 95°C for 10 minutes, followed by 40 cycles (45 cycles for downregulated genes) of denaturation at 95°C for 15 seconds, annealing at 60°C and extension at 60°C for 1 minute. A control human RNA (Stratagene, La Jolla, CA) was used for generating standard curves for ß-actin (internal standard) and target genes by plotting Ct-values versus template copy numbers. The copy number of each target gene was normalised to that of the housekeeping gene ß-actin using standard curves. The expression of each candidate gene was calculated as the ratio of the expression of that gene in cell lines with *B-RAF* and *N-RAS* mutations or homozygous deletion of *CDKN2A* to those in cell lines carrying no mutation or deletion.

3.4.2. *Determination of expression levels of B-RAF, N-RAS and CDKN2A in melanoma cell lines*

Expression levels of B-RAF, N-RAS and CDKN2A mRNA were determined in 97 melanoma cell lines from 97 individuals. Of the 97 cell lines, 50 (51%) carried mutations in the *B-RAF* gene, 24 (25%) had mutations in *N-RAS* and 33 (34%) had homozygous deletion of the *CDKN2A* gene (see results section 4.1.). cDNA synthesis from 1 µg of total RNA from the cell lines was carried out as described above. TaqMan Gene Expression Assays (Applied Biosystems, Foster City, CA) were used for detection of mRNA levels of B-RAF, N-RAS and CDKN2A (detection of both p16 and p14). Real-time PCR assay was performed as described under 3.4.1..

Expression of the target genes (*B-RAF*, *N-RAS* and *CDKN2A*) was compared with expression of the reference gene (β-actin), without use of a standard curve. Therefore, a validation experiment was performed to demonstrate optimal and identical real-time amplification efficiencies of target and reference genes. For every sample an equalisation of the Ct-values observed from the reference gene was done by multiplication with an "equalisation factor". With this process all samples were brought up to a common initial Ct-value and were comparable to each other in a collective analysis (personal communication; M. Hummel, Pathology, Campus Benjamin Franklin, Charité, Berlin).

Data analyses were performed using SAS software (SAS Institute, Cary, NC; version 9.13). Logistic regression analysis was performed to investigate the relationship between response variables and a set of explanatory variables. Response variables include the mRNA expression levels of B-RAF, N-RAS and CDKN2A. Explanatory variables include the mutational status of those genes. Odds ratios with accompanying 95% confidence intervals were calculated using maximum-likelihood estimates from multivariate and stepwise logistic regression models to describe the association of each explanatory variable with mRNA expression levels of B-RAF, N-RAS and CDKN2A. Continuous and ordinal variables were categorized for the analysis, to enable visualization of any nonlinear trends. Linear trend was analyzed using the Wald test by modeling each variable as a single continuous covariate. For continuous variables, the trend test was performed, using the median value within each category as the category score. All tests of statistical significance employed an α level of 0.05.

3.4.3. Determination of the AKAP9-B-RAF fusion transcript in melanoma cell lines

cDNA synthesised from total RNA was used for detection of the oncogenic AKAP9 - B-RAF fusion transcript in the melanoma cell lines. cDNA synthesis was carried out as described above. Primers designed had binding sites located in exon 8 of *AKAP9* (Ex8AKAP, 5´-AAG TAA GCA AGA ACA GTT GAT-3´) and exon 10 of *B-RAF* (Ex10BRAF, 5´-AAG CTT TCA CGT TAG TTA GT-3´) with an expected product length of 233 bp. A plasmid with full-length AKAP9 – B-RAF cDNA was used as a control kindly provided by Prof. Yuri Nikiforov, Department of Pathology, University of Cincinnati, USA. Integrity of the cDNA was controlled in selected cell lines by amplification of the housekeeping gene glycerinaldehyd-3-phosphat-dehydrogenase *(GAPDH)*. The primers used for amplification of the *GAPDH* fragment (209 bp) were forward 5´-GCA TCC TGGGCT ACA CTG AG-3´, and reverse 5´-GGT GGT CCA GGG GTC TTA CTC-3´. Genomic DNA from lymphocytes from healthy individuals were used as a control for amplification of cDNA.

PCR was performed in a 20 µl reaction mixture containing 1 ng cDNA from melanoma cell lines and 10 ng control genomic DNA from lymphocytes, respectively, 1 x PCR buffer, 2 mM magnesium chloride, 0.11 mM of each dNTP (Invitrogen, Paisley, UK), 0.3 µM forward and reverse primer, respectively (MWG Biotech AG, Ebersberg, Germany), 0.8 U Platinum Taq Polymerase (Invitrogen) and dH$_2$O. The PCR was carried out on a GeneAmp 9700 PCR System (Applied Biosystems, Foster City, USA). Initial denaturation was performed at 94°C for 1 minute, followed by 35 cycles each consisting of denaturation at 94°C for 30 seconds, annealing at 53°C

(59°C for PCR with the *GAPDH* primers) for 30 seconds and extension at 72°C for 30 seconds. Final extension was at 72°C for 5 minutes. 5 µl of the PCR products were subsequently analysed on a 1% agarose gel (Sigma, Munich, Germany), stained by ethidium bromide, which was run at a constant voltage of 120V in 1 x TAE (40 mM Tris acetate, 1 mM EDTA) for 20 minutes. DNA bands were visualized using a UV Bio Imaging System (Syngene, Cambridge, UK).

4. RESULTS

4.1. Mutations in the B-RAF and N-RAS genes and alterations of the CDKN2A gene locus in melanoma cell lines

In a panel of 140 melanoma cell lines (106 individuals) we detected mutations in exons 11 and 15 of the *B-RAF* gene in 81 (58%) cell lines (58 individuals) and mutually exclusive mutations in exons 1 and 2 of the *N-RAS* gene in 31 (22%) cell lines (28 individuals). Only one cell line carried mutations in both *B-RAF* and *N-RAS* genes. As shown in Table 7, five different *B-RAF* mutations were identified. The most common mutation was T1799A detected in 69/140 (49%) cell lines (51 patients). This mutation causes an amino acid change from valine to glutamic acid at codon 600 (V600E) in exon 15. Five patients (5%) carried the GT1798-99AA mutation at codon 600 (V600K) (Figure 10). Only two mutations in exon 15 were non-600; D594N and L597R, found in one patient each. In five cell lines from a single patient a GGA to AGA substitution (G469R) in exon 11 of *B-RAF* was detected.

Mutations in the *N-RAS* gene mostly occurred in codon 61 of exon 2 and were present in 28/140 (20%) cell lines (25 patients) (Table 7). The most common mutation was the CAA to CGA transition, causing a amino acid change from glutamine to arginine (Q61R) (Figure 10). This mutation was detected in 18/140 (13%) cell lines (15 individuals). In 8 (6%) cell lines (8 patients) a CAA to AAA transversion was detected, resulting in a glutamine to lysine change in amino acid (Q61K). Moreover, a CAA to CTA substitution, resulting in a glutamine to leucine exchange (Q61L), was detected in two cell lines obtained from the same individual. In addition to the mutation in codon 61 (Q61K), one patient carried a second *N-RAS* mutation at codon 68 (R68T). Mutations in exon 1 at codons 12 and 13 of the *N-RAS* gene were detected in 4 cell lines (4 individuals). A G13D and G13R amino acid change was identified in one patient each.

In a follow-up study in our laboratory, homozygous deletion of the *CDKN2A* locus was detected in 51 (41 individuals) out of 140 (36%) melanoma cell lines. Out of 81 cell lines with *B-RAF* mutation 38 (47%) additionally showed homozygous deletion of the *CDKN2A* locus. Similarly, of the 32 cell lines with *N-RAS* mutation 9 (27%) had homozygous deletion at the *CDKN2A* locus. Thus, out of 112 cell lines (80 individuals) with either *B-RAF* or *N-RAS* mutations, 46 (41%) cell lines (37 individuals) also had homozygous deletion at the *CDKN2A* locus. Conversely, out of 28 cell lines

(23 individuals) without *B-RAF* or *N-RAS* mutation only 5 (4 individuals) showed homozygous deletion at the *CDKN2A* locus.

Table 7. Mutations in *B-RAF* and *N-RAS* genes in melanoma cell lines.

	Cell lines 140 (100%)	Patients 106 (100%)
B-RAF mutation	81 (58)	58 (55)
Exon 11	**5 (4)**	**1 (1)**
G469R	5 (4)	1 (1)
Exon 15	**76 (54)**	**58 (55)**
V600E	69 (49)	51 (48)
V600K	5 (4)	5 (5)
D594N*	1 (1)	1 (1)
L597R	1 (1)	1 (1)
N-RAS mutation	32 (23)	28 (26)
Exon 1	**4 (2)**	**4 (4)**
G12D	2 (1)	2 (2)
G13D*	1 (1)	1 (1)
G13R	1 (1)	1 (1)
Exon 2	**28 (20)**	**24 (23)**
Q61R	18 (13)	15 (14)
Q61K**	8 (6)	8 (7)
Q61L	2 (1)	1 (1)
B-RAF or N-RAS mutation	**111 (79)**	**79 (74)**
*B-RAF **and** N-RAS* mutation in the same cell line*	**1 (1)**	**1 (1)**
*B-RAF **and** N-RAS* mutation in different cell lines from the same individual	**9 (6)**	**3 (3)**
No B-RAF or *N-RAS* mutation	**28 (20)**	**23 (22)**

* one cell line with D594N mutation in *B-RAF* also carried a G13D mutation in *N-RAS*
** one cell line with Q61K *N-RAS* mutation had an additional R68T mutation in *N-RAS*

Taken together, our results showed a significant overlap between mutations in the *B-RAF/N-RAS* genes and homozygous deletions at the *CDKN2A* locus (OR 5.21, 95% CI 1.14-9.1, P=0.02).

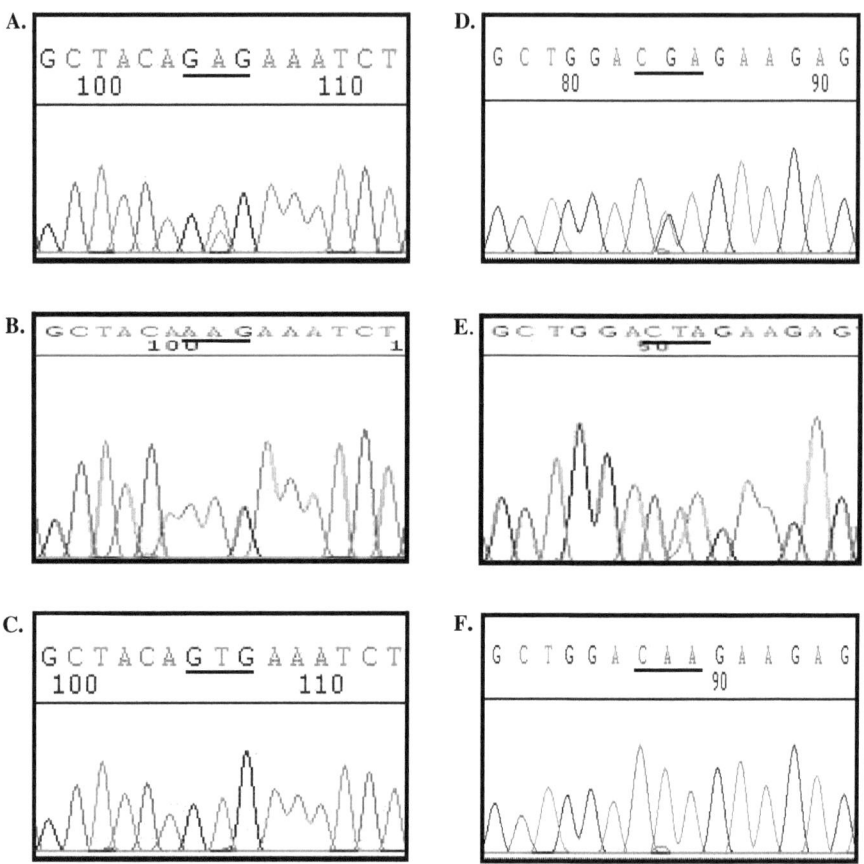

Figure 10. Sequence analysis of *B-RAF* and *N-RAS* genes. The left side of the picture presents parts of exon 15 of the *B-RAF* gene sequence showing A) T1799A base change (V600E), B) GT1798-99AA (V600K) tandem mutation, C) corresponding wild-type sequence. The right side of the figure shows parts of exon 2 of the *N-RAS* gene with D) A182G base change (Q61R), E) A182T base change (Q61L), F) corresponding wild-type sequence.

4.2. Levels of B-RAF, N-RAS and CDKN2A gene expression and correlation with mutations

Besides activating mutations, overexpression of B-RAF as a result of gene amplification has also been reported to be as one of the mechanisms leading to the activation of the MAPK pathway (242). Expression of three genes, *B-RAF, N-RAS* and *CDKN2A,* was determined by quantitative real-time PCR as described in "Materials and Methods". We correlated the expression with the mutational status of those genes in melanoma cell lines using logistic regression analysis (Table 8).

Data analysis showed that expression of B-RAF was significantly lower in melanoma cell lines with *N-RAS* mutations than in cell lines without such mutations (Table 8). The inverse relationship between *N-RAS* mutations and B-RAF expression implied positive correlation with *B-RAF* mutations. The statistical analysis showed increased expression of B-RAF in cell lines with *B-RAF* mutations. However, the relationship was not statistically significant (Table 8). No effect of *B-RAF* mutations on expression of N-RAS was observed. However, N-RAS expression was lower in cell lines with homozygous deletion of *CDKN2A* and the effect was independend of *B-RAF* and *N-RAS* mutational status. Moreover, as expected, cell lines with homozygous deletion of the *CDKN2A* gene lacked expression.

Table 8. Estimation of the effects of alterations in the *B-RAF, N-RAS* and *CDKN2A* genes on their expression in melanoma cell lines.

Mutational status and effect	Odds Ratio	95% Confidence Limits
Effect on B-RAF expression		
N-RAS mutations	0.37	0.16 - 0.84
B-RAF mutations	1.79	0.89 - 3.60
Effect on N-RAS expression		
CDKN2A deletion	0.01	0.003 - 0.04
Effect on CDKN2A expression		
CDKN2A deletion	<0.001	<0.001 - >999.9

4.3. The AKAP9-B-RAF fusion transcript in melanoma cell lines

Besides melanoma, the *B-RAF* gene is frequently mutated in thyroid cancer. However, recently a unique mode of activation of B-RAF in radiation-induced thyroid papillary carcinoma was reported. Chromosomal re-arrangement resulting in an in-frame fusion between *B-RAF* and *AKAP9* was detected in 11% of early radiation-associated tumours. The overexpression of B-RAF through this mechanism in the absence of mutations leads to downstream activation of the MAPK pathway (212). In order to determine a similar chromosomal re-arrangement we screened our melanoma cell lines included in this study for the AKAP9 – B-RAF fusion transcript. A plasmid with the full-lenght AKAP9 – B-RAF fusion transcript was used as a positive control. The quality of cDNA was controlled by amplification of the housekeeping gene glycerinaldehyd-3-phosphat-dehydrogenase (*GAPDH*). Our results from this experiment showed that the primers used were successful in amplification of the fusion transcript. The cDNA used was of sufficient quality as shown by the amplification of the housekeeping gene. However, in none of the melanoma cell lines we detected the AKAP9 – B-RAF fusion transcript (Figure 11).

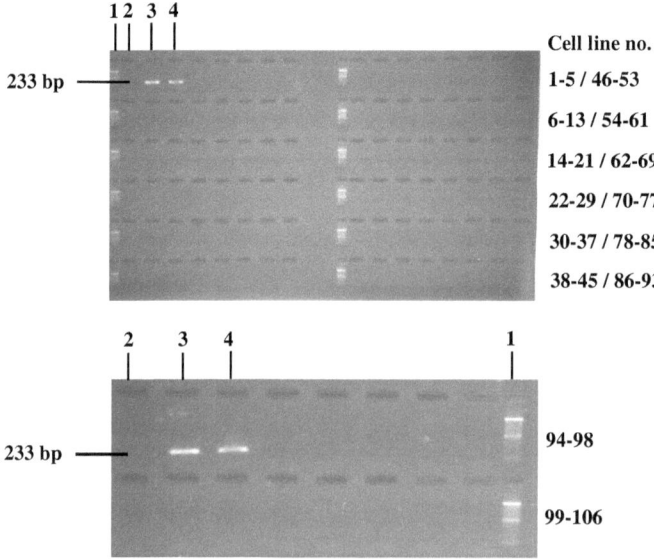

Figure 11. Screening of melanoma cell lines for the presence of the AKAP9 – B-RAF fusion transcript by agarose gel electrophoresis. Lanes 1: 100 bp DNA ladder (Invitrogen). Lanes 3 and 4 in both gel pictures show amplification from the plasmid containing the full-length fusion transcript as positive control. Lanes 2 were with negative control. None of the lanes with the amplification reaction from melanoma cell lines showed the presence of the fusion transcript. Amplification of *GAPDH* was used as positive control for cDNA.

4.4. Effect of V600E B-RAF and Q61R N-RAS mutations on global gene expression in melanoma cell lines

Three melanoma cell lines harbouring the V600E mutation in the *B-RAF* gene and four cell lines with the Q61R mutation in the *N-RAS* gene were analysed and compared with expression profiles of three melanoma cell lines without mutations in the *B-RAF* and *N-RAS* genes. None of the cell lines chosen for this study carried any genetic alterations in the *CDKN2A* gene. Three different softwares; GeneCip Operation Software (GCOS, Affymetrix), Significance Analysis of Microarrays (SAM) and GeneCluster2.0 were used to analyse the microarray data.

Results from microarray data analysed with GCOS

Expression analysis using the GCOS module showed that an average of 51% (11 380 ± 397.4) of transcripts were scored as being present in the cell lines harbouring the *B-RAF* mutation, an average of 53.7% (11 958 ± 78.1) of transcripts were present in cells containing the *N-RAS* mutation and an average of 52.4% (11 679 ± 96.5) of transcripts were present in cell lines without these mutations. Pair-wise comparison of expression data from each cell line with and without mutations was performed. From comparison with (3 cell lines from 3 individual patients) and without (3 cell lines from 3 individual patients) *B-RAF* mutation 9 data sets were obtained. Similarly, for 4 cell lines (from 4 individual patients) with *N-RAS* mutation and 3 cell lines (from 3 individual patients) without mutation 12 data sets were obtained.

Based on the criteria described under "Materials and Methods", 174 probe sets corresponding to 139 genes were found to be increased in cell lines with the *B-RAF* mutation and 211 probe sets (168 genes) were decreased when compared to cell lines without the mutations. Similarly, cell lines harbouring the *N-RAS* mutations showed a significant increase of 275 probe sets (203 genes) and a decrease of 208 probe sets (168 genes). The combination of data from cell lines with the *B-RAF* and *N-RAS* mutations showed an overlap of 86 probes (69 genes) upregulated in cell lines with these mutations as compared to cell lines without mutations. In comparison to cell lines without mutations 88 probes (70 genes) were increased specifically in *B-RAF* mutated cell lines and 189 probes (134 genes) were increased only in cell lines with *N-RAS* mutation. 112 probe sets (89 genes) showed an overlapping downregulation in cell lines with *B-RAF* and *N-RAS* mutations compared to cell lines without mutations. Similarly, in comparison to cell lines without mutations 99 probes (79 genes) were scored as decreased exclusively in cell lines with mutant *B-RAF* and 96 probes (79 genes) were found as significantly decreased only in cell lines with the *N-RAS* mutation.

Results from microarray data analysed with SAM

Using SAM for data analysis with a delta value of 1.05 and R=2 (2-fold change or more), as described in Material and Methods, 696 probes were called significant (169 positive corresponding to 146 genes, 527 negative corresponding to 467 genes) for cell lines carrying the *B-RAF* mutation when compared to cell lines without the mutation. This number of probes was well comparable to the 174 positively and 211 negatively changed probes identified by DMT. However, the data set yielded an estimated false discovery rate of 18.5%, which equals to an average of 129 falsely significant genes. After normalisation of signal values from cell lines with *N-RAS* mutation and those without mutation and data analysis using SAM with a delta of 1.59 (including the criteria of '2-fold or more change'), 767 probes (307 positive corresponding to 243 genes / 460 negative corresponding to 396 genes) were called significant with 7.3% false discovery rate corresponding to 56 genes.

Data from marker analysis using GeneCluster2.0

For analysis of the microarray data using GeneCluster2.0 filter criteria as described in "Materials and Methods" were used. For the cell lines with mutant *B-RAF*, 4546 probes passed these filters and for cell lines with the *N-RAS* mutation 4279 probes passed these criteria. Supervised analysis of the data demonstrated a clear separation of the cell lines with the V600E *B-RAF* mutation from the cell lines with Q61R *N-RAS* mutation. Figure 12 shows a set of 20 best correlated markers which are distinct for each group of cell lines. A number of genes, among those various members of the MAPK pathway, distinguish cell lines with either *B-RAF* or *N-RAS* mutations and cell lines without any mutations. Figure 13 displays a set of 30 best correlated markers that separate cell lines with either *B-RAF* or *N-RAS* mutations from cell lines without any mutations. For the purpose of further comparisons of the probe lists and the identification of overlapping probe sets between cell lines with mutations we chose the first 300 increased/decreased probe sets.

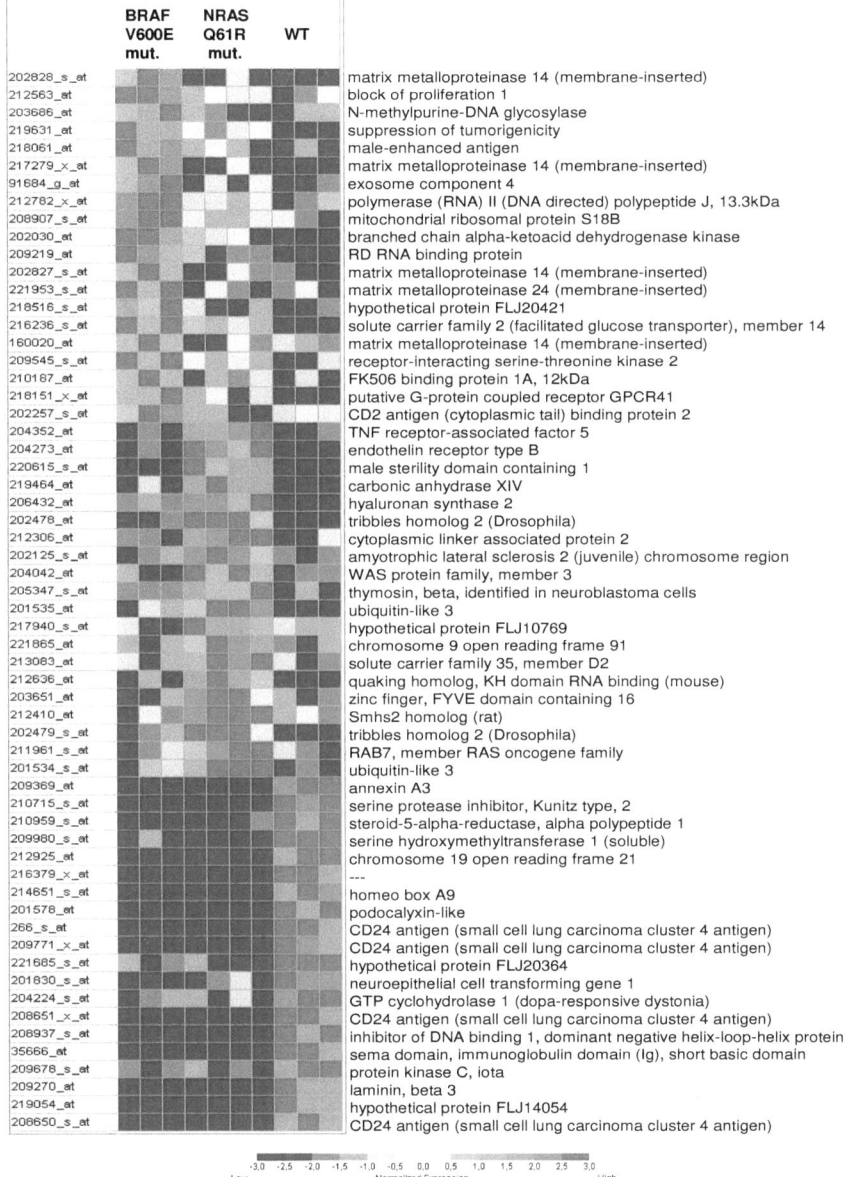

Figure 12. Results from a marker gene analysis showing 20 best correlated genes with differential expressions in cell lines with *B-RAF* mutation, *N-RAS* mutation and cell lines without mutations. Markers were selected by computing the Signal to Noise score. The columns shown represent individual samples and rows represent single genes and are ranked in a `best-correlated` order. The colour scale identifies relative gene expression changes normalised by the standard deviation, with 0 representing the mean expression level of a given gene across the panel.

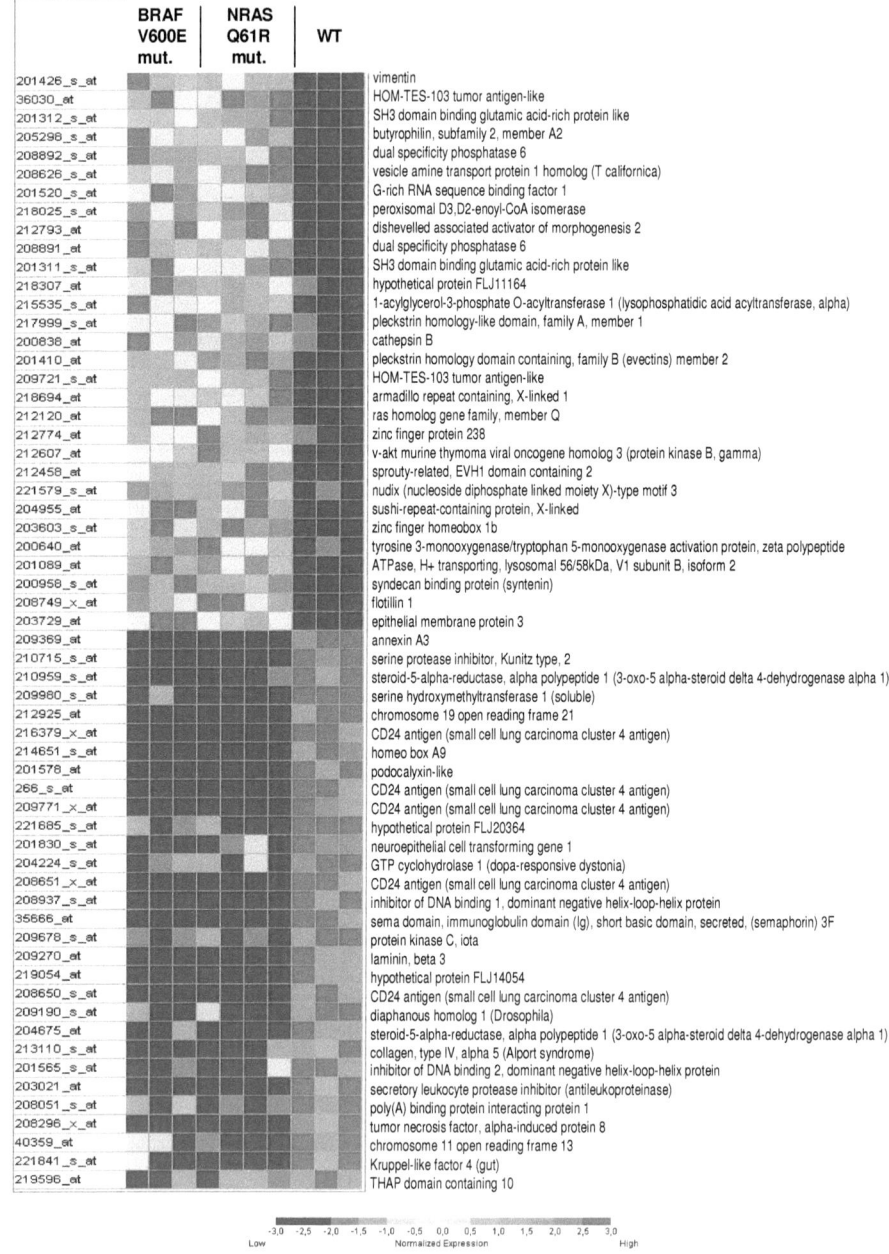

Figure 13. Results from a marker gene analysis of microarray data with 30 best correlated genes in cell lines with *B-RAF* and *N-RAS* mutations compared with cell lines with no mutations.

Combination of the data obtained from the three software modules
In order to increase the stringency of data analysis, the list of genes obtained from the three software modules were combined (Figure 14, Tables 9 and 10). In cell lines with the *B-RAF* mutation 40 genes were found to be significantly upregulated (Figure 14A) and 77 genes were significantly downregulated (Figure 14B) when compared to the cell lines containing no such mutations. Similar comparison showed that in cell lines with the *N-RAS* mutation 81 genes were with significantly increased expression (Figure 14C) and 84 genes with decreased expression (Figure 14D). We found that 11 genes were significantly increased in cell lines with *B-RAF* and *N-RAS* mutations relative to cell lines without mutations (Figure 14E). 70 genes appeared to be upregulated specifically in cell lines with the *N-RAS* mutation, 29 genes were markedly upregulated only in cell lines with the *B-RAF* mutation (Figure 14E and Appendix, Table 9). Similarly, 45 genes were downregulated in cell lines with the *B-RAF* and *N-RAS* mutations, 32 genes were specific to cell lines with the *B-RAF* mutations and 39 specific to cell lines with *N-RAS* mutations (Figure 14F and Appendix, Table 10).

Some of the genes which showed a distinctive overexpression in cell lines with mutations in *B-RAF* and *N-RAS* genes in comparison to the cell lines without mutations included dual-specificity phosphatase 6 (*DUSP6*), v-akt murine thymoma viral oncogene homolog 3 (*AKT3*) and sprouty homolog 2 (*SPRY2*). In cell lines with mutations against cell lines without mutations interleukin 18 (*IL18*), tumor necrosis factor, alpha-induced protein 8 (*TNFAIP8*), inhibitor of DNA binding (*ID2*) and Krüppel-like factors 4 and 5 (*KLF4* and *5*) were downregulated. Besides others, genes that were overexpressed only in cell lines with *N-RAS* mutations included melan-A (*MLANA*), glutathione S-transferase M1 and M4 (*GSTM1* and *4*), Ras-related GTP binding D (*RRAGD*) and dual-specificity phosphatase 4 (*DUSP4*). Matrix metalloproteinase 14 (*MMP14*), *FYN* oncogene and melanoma antigen, family A, 3 (*MAGEA3*) were among the genes observed to be upregulated specifically in cell lines harboring mutation in the *B-RAF* gene in comparison to cell lines without mutations.

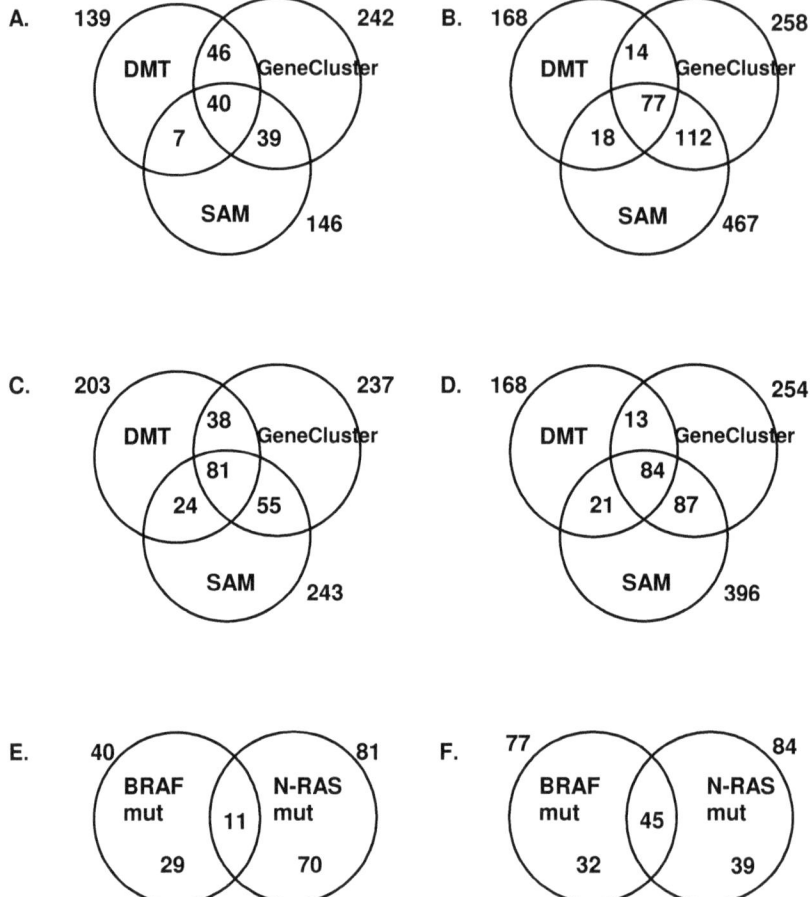

Figure 14. Venn diagram representing the number of genes that showed differential expression in melanoma cell lines with *B-RAF* and *N-RAS* mutations compared to cell lines without mutations after evaluation of microarray data with three different softwares (see: Materials and Methods). **A:** number of upregulated genes in cell lines with *B-RAF* mutation as shown by three different softwares; **B:** downregulated genes in cell lines with *B-RAF* mutation; **C:** number of genes with relative increased expression in cell lines with *N-RAS* mutation; **D:** decreased expression of genes in cell lines with *N-RAS* mutation; **E:** Filtered data from **1A-D** showing the number of common and specific genes upregulated in cell lines with *B-RAF* and *N-RAS* mutations and **F:** the number of common and specific genes downregulated in cell lines with *B-RAF* and *N-RAS* mutations.

Validation of microarray data

For a selected group of genes real-time PCR was used to validate the microarray expression data (Table 6 in "Materials and Methods"). The criteria for gene inclusion in real-time PCR experiments were their potential role in melanocyte biology, the MAPK pathway or cell cycle regulation. Our results from real-time PCR confirmed the microarray data for all the selected genes. In microarray experiments *DUSP6* showed an 8-fold overexpression in cell lines with mutations in the *B-RAF* and *N-RAS* genes relative to the cell lines without mutations and in real-time PCR experiments in a similar comparison isoform 'a' of *DUSP6* showed a 12-fold overexpression (Figure 15.1.A); isoform b showed only 2-fold upregulation (data not shown). The overexpression of *TAZ*, *SPRY2* and *AKT3* observed in microarray experiments in cell lines with the mutations compared to cell lines without mutations were confirmed by RT-PCR (Figures 15.1.B-D). The expression results from real-time PCR for *MMP14* were in agreement with microarray data, which showed 4.5 and 4.6-fold increase, respectively in cell lines with mutation in the *B-RAF* gene compared to cell without mutations (Figure 15.1.E). However, in real-time experiments *MMP14* was also shown to be slightly overexpressed in cell lines with the *N-RAS* mutation (Figure 15.1.E). Microarray data for *TAZ* and *SPRY2* genes showed overexpression only in cell lines with the *B-RAF* mutations (Appendix, Table 9), however, in the real-time experiments both genes were confirmed as upregulated in all cell lines with the *B-RAF* and *N-RAS* mutation compared to cell lines with no mutations. In microarray data analysis the filter was set for inclusion of probe sets with a signal log ratio of 1, which being 0.99 for *TAZ* and *SPRY2* genes in cell lines with *N-RAS* mutations resulted in their exclusion from the list of overexpressed genes.

Similarly, underexpression of *ID2* seen in microarray experiments (4.8-fold) was confirmed for all cell lines harbouring mutations in the *B-RAF* and *N-RAS* genes in real-time PCR experiments (4.6-fold, Figure 15.2.F). *PDCD4* was confirmed to be more drastically downregulated in cell lines with the mutant *B-RAF* (microarray 5.3-fold/real time-PCR 5.7-fold) than in cell lines harbouring the *N-RAS* mutation (microarray 1.7-fold/real-time PCR 1.9-fold, Figure 15.2.G) when compared over all to the cell lines without mutations. *IL18* and *KLF5* expression was totally repressed in cell lines with mutations, more so in cell lines with *B-RAF* mutations than in cell lines with *N-RAS* mutations (Figures 15.2.H and I).

A. DUSP6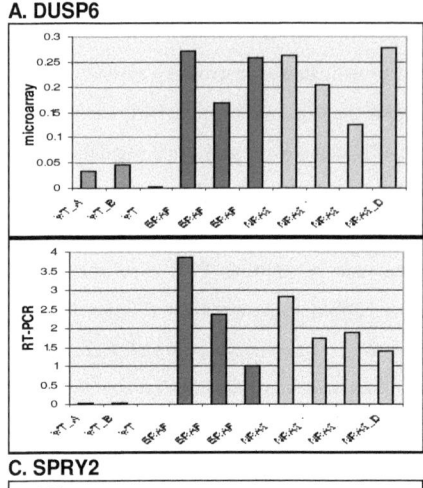

B. AKT3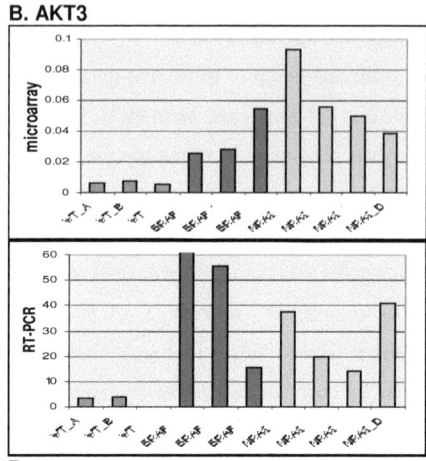

C. SPRY2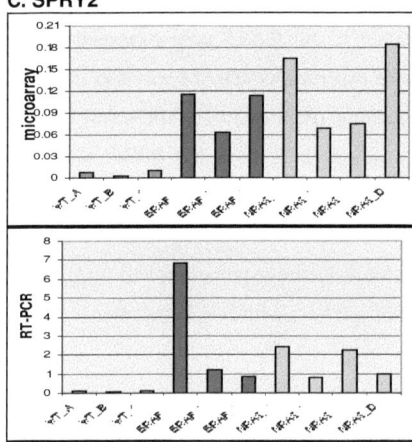

D. TAZ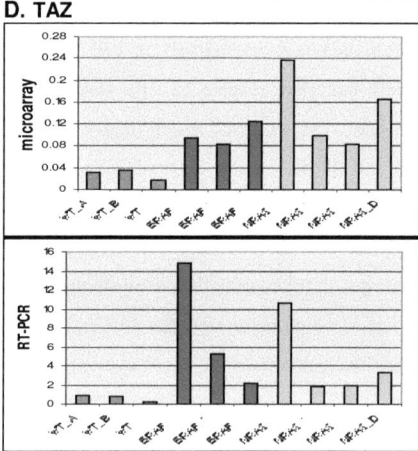

E. MMP14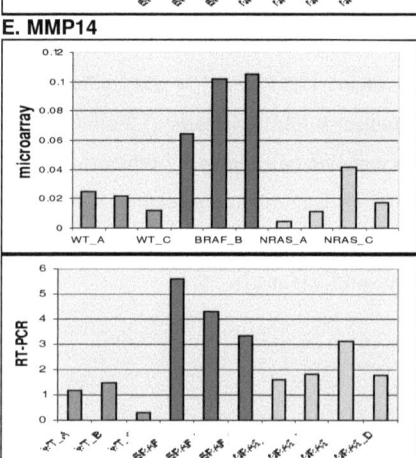

Figure 15.1. Validation of the microarray results with real-time PCR technique. **A-E**: Panels show level of upregulation of genes from microarray data (upper panels) and from RT-PCR data (lower panels); WT_A-C represent three cell lines without mutations; BRAF_A-C three cell lines with V600E mutation in the *B-RAF* gene and NRAS_A-D four cell lines with Q61R mutation in the *N-RAS* gene. The Y-axis in upper panel in A-E represents microarray signals normalised to β-actin and in lower panel Y-axis represents real-time PCR signal intensity normalised to β-actin.

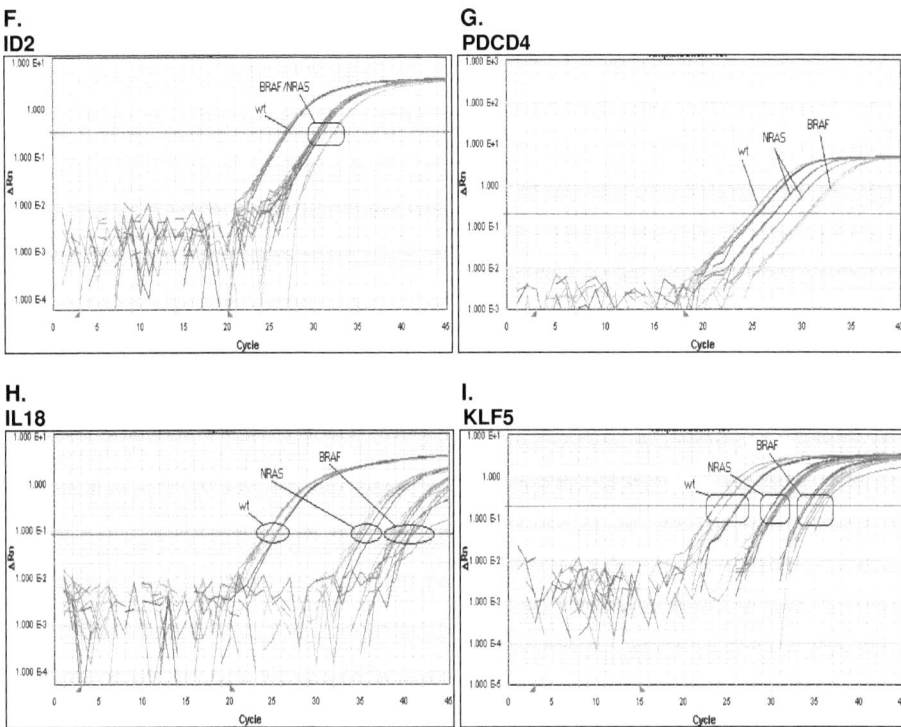

Figure 15.2. Validation of the microarray results with real-time PCR technique. **F-I**: Panels show real-time amplification plots of four genes that showed downregulation in microarray experiments in cell lines with mutations in the *B-RAF* and *N-RAS* genes compared to cell lines without mutation.

4.5. Differences in global gene expression in melanoma cell lines with and without homozygous deletions of the CDKN2A locus genes

Four melanoma cell lines with and three cell lines without homozygous deletion of the *CDKN2A* locus (including the *CDKN2B* gene) for comparison of expression profiles using Affymetrix oligonucleotide arrays were selected. None of the cell lines selected for expression analysis carried mutations in the *B-RAF* and *N-RAS* genes. Microarray data were analysed with 3 different softwares; GCOS, SAM and GeneCluster2.0. The results of differential expression in cell lines with and without homozygous deletions of the *CDKN2A* gene were compared with data from cell lines with *B-RAF* and *N-RAS* mutations described under 4.4..

Results from analysis of microarray data with GCOS
Expression analysis with GCOS module showed an average of 51.1% (11 385 ± 280.8) transcripts as present in samples with and an average of 52.4% (11 679 ± 96.5) transcripts present in samples without a *CDKN2A* deletion. Pair-wise comparison of expression data from each cell line with (4 cell lines) and without (3 cell lines) *CDKN2A* deletion were performed yielding 12 data sets. Data were sorted in DMT according to the criteria described under "Materials and Methods". Based on these criteria 234 probe sets corresponding to 169 genes had increased expression in cell lines with the *CDKN2A* deletion and 222 probe sets (169 genes) were correspondingly decreased.

Results from analysis of microarray data using SAM
Analysis of microarray data using SAM revealed 1260 probes that were significantly changed. 301 probes corresponding to 238 genes were significantly increased and 959 probes corresponding to 752 genes were decreased in cell lines lacking the *CDKN2A* gene. The estimated false discovery rate was 12.9 %.

Results from marker gene analysis using GeneCluster2.0
4382 transcripts showed differential regulation in cell lines with *CDKN2A* deletion relative to cell lines without deletion. In further comparisons with results from the two other software modules the first 300 increased/decreased probe sets representing 234 and 253 genes with increased and decreased expression in the cell lines were chosen.

Combination of the data from the three software modules
In order to increase the stringency of the analysis of microarray data, the probe lists obtained from the three software modules were combined. From this combination, 70 genes with increased

expression and 86 genes with decreased expression were found in cell lines with *CDKN2A* homozygous deletion (Figures 16A and 16B). Genes involved in disparate pathways showed relative up- and downregulation (Appendix, Tables 11 and 12). Most prominently upregulated genes in the cell lines with deletion included calpain 3 (*CAPN3*, 653-fold), peroxisomal D3,D2-enoyl-CoA isomerase (*PECI*, 274-fold), vimentin (*VIM*, 148-fold), tyrosinase (*TYR*, 71-fold), endothelin receptor type B (*EDNRB*, 105-fold) and melanoma antigen, family A, member 2, 6, and 12 (*MAGE A2*, 128-fold; *MAGEA6*, 623-fold and *MAGEA12*, 90-fold) (Appendix, Table 11). Amongst the downregulated genes in the cell lines with homozygous deletion were interleukin 18 (*IL18*, 489-fold), inhibitor of DNA binding 2 (*ID2*, 3-fold), Krüppel-like factor 4 (*KLF4*, 9-fold), CD24 antigen (*CD24*, 1308-fold) and others (Appendix, Table 12).

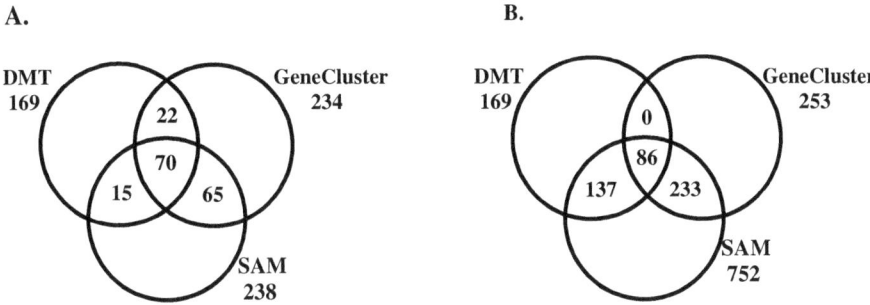

Figure 16. Venn diagram representing the number of genes with changes in the expression after evaluation of the microarray data with the three different softwares DMT, SAM and GeneCluster2.0 (see: Materials and Methods); **A.** number of upregulated genes in cell lines with *CDKN2A* homozygous deletion; and **B.** down-regulated genes in cell lines with *CDKN2A* deletion.

Results of gene ontology analysis using the Gene Ontology Mining Tool (Affymetrix)

In order to obtain a statistical estimate about the over-representation of genes related to a specific biological process microarray data were applied to the Gene Ontology Mining Tool. The results showed over-representation of various genes involved in cellular metabolism and protein modification. Of the 70 genes which we found significantly upregulated, 22 mapped to development processes (X^2 18.5, P<0.0001). Some of the genes in this pathway included sprouty homolog 2 and 4 (*SPRY2* and *4*), laminin, α-4 (*LAMA4*), calpain 3 (*CAPN3*), endothelial receptor type B (*EDNRB*), down syndrome critical region gene 1 (*DSCR1*), dopachrome tautomerase (*DCT*) and tyrosinase (*TYR*). Of the 19 upregulated genes involved in cell communication, 4 regulated signal transduction (X^2 8.5, P 0.004), which included sprouty homolog 2 and 4 (*SPRY2* and *4*) and extra-cellular matrix protein 1 (*ECM1*). Analysis of 86 downregulated genes showed 54 genes in cellular processes (X^2 6.5, P 0.01). 45 genes were involved in cellular physiological processes (X^2 3.9, P 0.08) and out of those 9 in cell proliferation (X^2 9.0, P 0.003). The genes involved in cell proliferation included ryanodine receptor 1 (*RYR1*), interleukin 18 (*IL18*), Krüppel-like factor 4 (*KLF4*) and stratifin (*SFN*). 28 downregulated genes included those involved in cellular metabolism (X^2 5.8, P 0.02), which included one gene adenosine kinase (*ADK*) in the metabolic compound salvage pathway (X^2 39.1, P<0.0001).

Results of pathway analysis using the Ingenuity Pathways Analysis 3.0 Software
In order to map our set of differentially expressed gene to known functions and pathways microarray data were also analysed by the Ingenuity Pathways Analysis 3.0 Software (Ingenuity Systems, Inc., Redwood City, CA). Out of 156 significantly differentially expressed genes (70 up-, 86 downregulated) in cell lines with *CDKN2A* deletion, 112 genes could be mapped to known pathways and functions. 77 were known to have relevant functions or were linked to diseases. Out of those 77 genes, 43 were involved in cell death and cell invasion. Such genes included vimentin (*VIM*, 148-fold upregulation), secreted protein acidic and rich in cysteine (*SPARC*, 383-fold upregulation), dopachrome tautomerase (*DCT*, 42-fold upregulation), tyrosinase (*TYR*, 71-fold upregulation), endothelin receptor type B (*EDNRB*, 105-fold upregulation), integrin, beta 3 (*ITGB3*, 28-fold upregulation), S-phase kinase-associated protein 2 (*SKP2*, 7-fold downregulation), inhibitors of DNA binding 1 and 2 (*ID1*, 32-fold downregulation; *ID2*, 3-fold downregulation) and dual specificity phosphatases 1 and 6 (*DUSP1*, 7-fold downregulation; *DUSP6*, 67-fold upregulation). 37 genes were involved in apoptosis, which included homeo box A9 (*HOXA9*, 45-fold downregulated) and SRY (sex determining region Y)-box 10 (*SOX10*, 36-fold upregulated). 24 genes, including tyrosinase and dopachrome tautomerase, exerted functions in melanin biosynthesis. 23 genes acted in cellular growth and proliferation, which included interleukin 18 (*IL18*) and secreted protein acidic and rich in cysteine (*SPARC*).

Comparison of differential gene expression in cell lines with and without alterations in the B-RAF, N-RAS and CDKN2A genes
Differential gene expression in cell lines with homozygous deletion of the *CDKN2A* gene was compared with our earlier differential expression data from cell lines with *B-RAF* and *N-RAS* mutations. In marker analysis, microarray data revealed a distinct set of probes that clustered cell lines with mutations in the *B-RAF/N-RAS* genes and homozygous deletion of the *CDKN2A* gene separately from melanoma cell lines without alterations in any of these genes. The genes that

showed overlapping upregulation in cell lines with *B-RAF/N-RAS* mutations and *CDKN2A* deletion included *AKT3, DUSP6, SPRY2, VIM* and others. The downregulated genes common to cell lines with alterations included *CD24*, Kunitz type 2 serine protease inhibitor (*SPINT2*), *KLF4,* and protein kinase C (*PRKCI*). With combination of differential expression data an overlapping upregulation of 7 genes and downregulation of 23 genes were found in cell lines with *B-RAF* and *N-RAS* mutations or *CDKN2A* homozygous deletion compared to cell lines without alteration in these genes (Table 13).

Table 13. Comparison of differential gene expression in cell lines with and without alterations in *B-RAF*, *N-RAS* and *CDKN2A* genes using three different software modules. Upregulated and downregulated genes common in cell lines with V600E *B-RAF* /Q61R *N-RAS* mutation or homozygous deletion of *CDKN2A* compared to cell lines without alterations in those genes.

Gene Name	Gene Symbol
7 Increased genes	
SH3 domain binding glutamic acid-rich protein like	SH3BGRL
vimentin	VIM
solute carrier family 2 (facilitated glucose transporter), member 3	SLC2A3
vesicle amine transport protein 1 homolog (T californica)	VAT1
v-akt murine thymoma viral oncogene homolog 3 (protein kinase B, gamma)	AKT3
dual specificity phosphatase 6	DUSP6
HOM-TES-103 tumor antigen-like	HOM-TES-103
23 Decreased genes	
annexin A3	ANXA3
CD24 antigen (small cell lung carcinoma cluster 4 antigen)	CD24
chromosome 19 open reading frame 21	C19orf21
coagulation factor III (thromboplastin, tissue factor)	F3
GTP cyclohydrolase 1 (dopa-responsive dystonia)	GCH1
homeo box A9	HOXA9
hypothetical protein FLJ14054	FLJ14054
inhibitor of DNA binding 1, dominant negative helix-loop-helix protein	ID1
keratin 17	KRT17
keratin 8	KRT8
Kruppel-like factor 4 (gut)	KLF4
laminin, beta 3	LAMB3
myosin VC	MYO5C
neuroepithelial cell transforming gene 1	NET1
podocalyxin-like	PODXL
secretory leukocyte protease inhibitor (antileukoproteinase)	SLPI
sema domain, immunoglobulin domain (Ig), short basic domain, secreted, 3F	SEMA3F
serine protease inhibitor, Kunitz type, 2	SPINT2
solute carrier family 29 (nucleoside transporters), member 3	SLC29A3
steroid-5-alpha-reductase, alpha polypeptide 1 (3-oxo-5 alpha-steroid delta 4-dehydrogenase alpha 1)	SRD5A1
THAP domain containing 10	THAP10
tuftelin 1	TUFT1
tumor necrosis factor, alpha-induced protein 8	TNFAIP8

Validation of microarray data

The absence and presence of the CDKN2A mRNA expression in cell lines with and without homozygous deletion of the *CDKN2A* gene was confirmed using quantitative real-time PCR (data not shown). Furthermore, the results from microarray data for four genes with increased expression and four genes with decreased expression in cell lines with the deletion compared to cell lines without deletions was confirmed. The genes that were selected for validation of microarray data with real-time PCR were *DUSP6*, *AKT3*, *SPRY2* and *TAZ* for relative upregulation and *IL18*, *ID2*, *KLF5* and *PDCD4* for relative downregulation (Table 6 in "Materials and Methods"). For all the transcripts studied by real-time PCR data were in concordance with microarray data (Figures 17a and 17b).

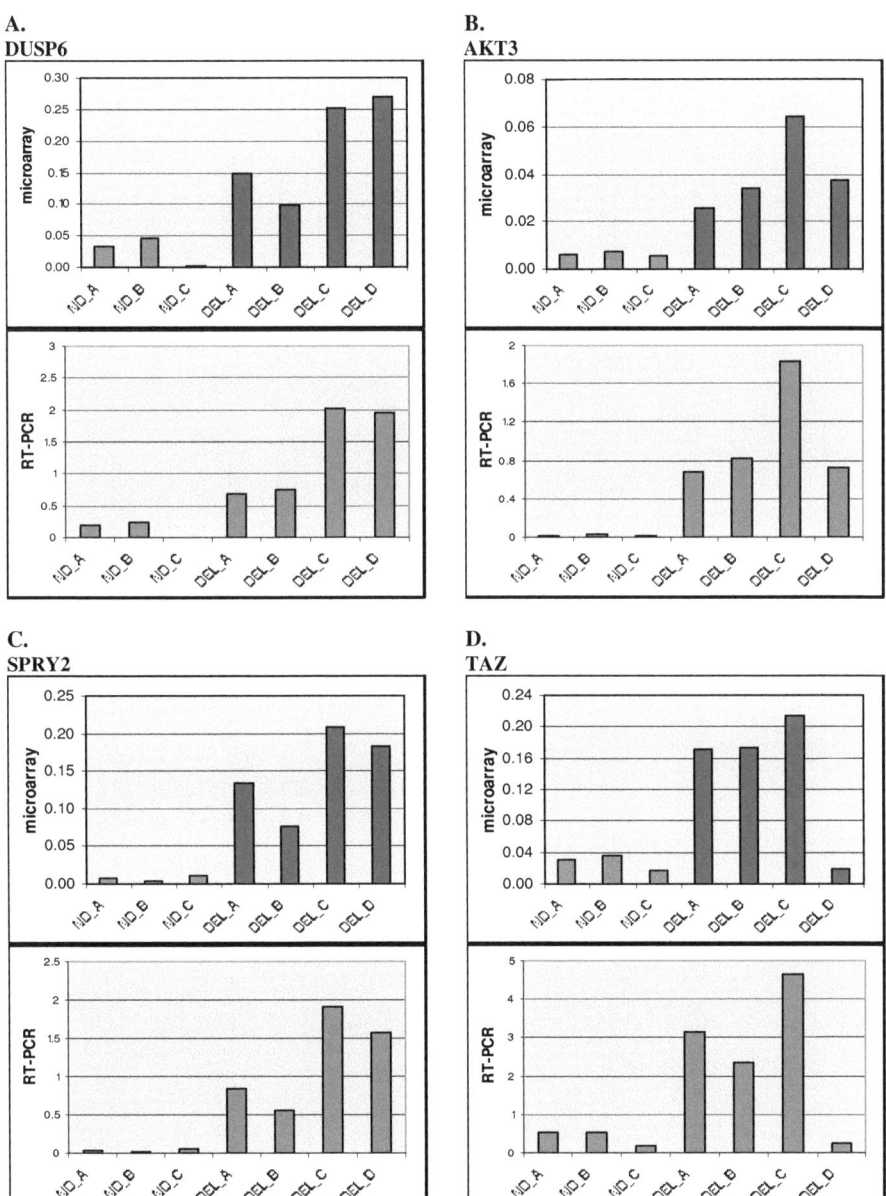

Figure 17a. The results from microarray experiments for selected genes were validated with real-time PCR technique. **A-D** panels showing level of upregulation of genes from microarray data (**upper panels**) and from RT-PCR data (**lower panels**) ND_A-C represent three cell lines without homozygous deletions; DEL_A-D four cell lines with homozygous deletion of the *CDKN2A* gene.

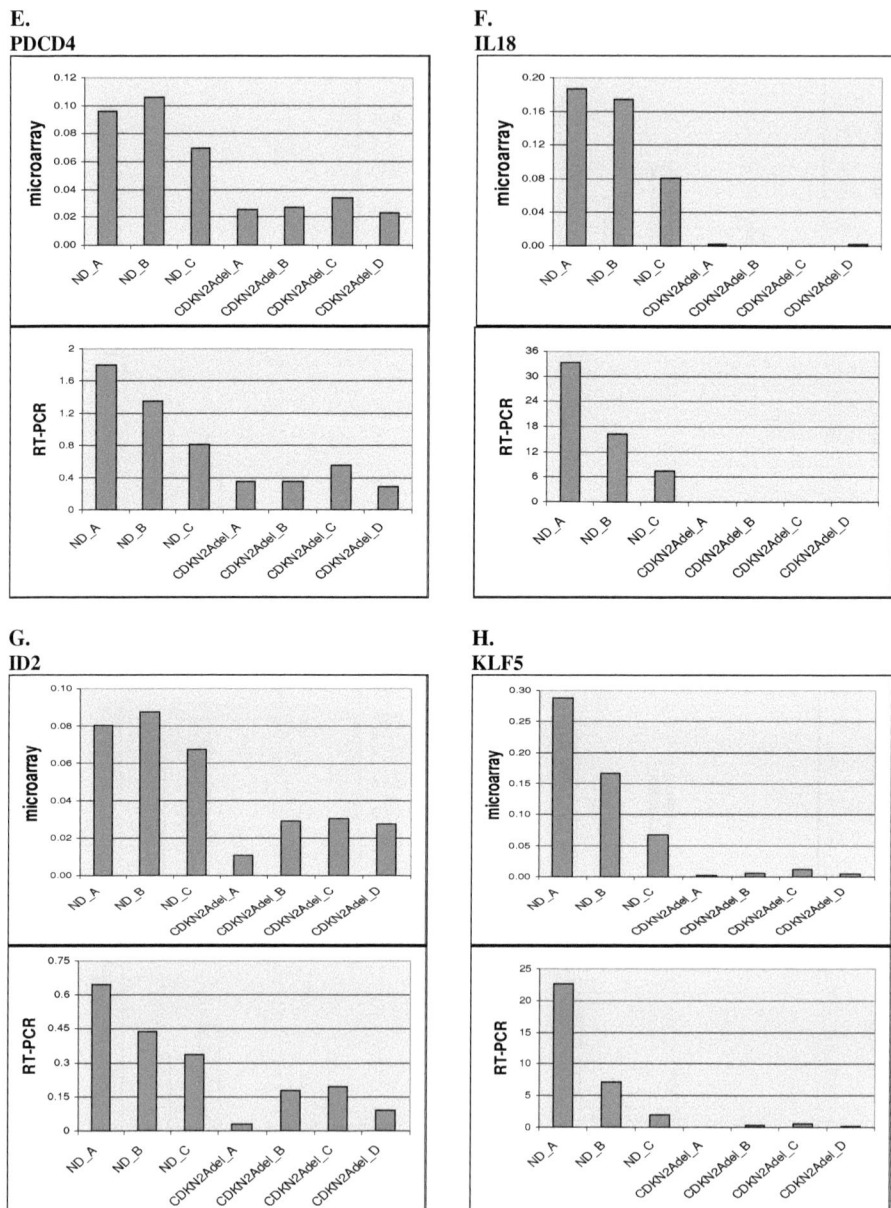

Figure 17b. The results from microarray experiments for selected genes were validated with real-time PCR technique. **E-H** panels showing level of downregulation from microarray data (**upper panels**) and from RT-PCR data (**lower panels**) ND_A-C represent three cell lines without homozygous deletions; CDKN2Adel_A-D four cell lines with homozygous deletion of the *CDKN2A* gene.

4.6. Effect of the V600E B-RAF mutation on global gene expression in melanocytic nevi

Thirty benign melanocytic nevi from ten individuals were screened for mutations in the *B-RAF* and *N-RAS* genes. 23 of the nevi from 9 individuals carried mutations in *B-RAF*. Two nevi from one individual carried *N-RAS* mutations (Q61K and Q61R), while three more nevi from the same individual showed the V600E *B-RAF* mutation. From two individuals from whom three and four nevi were screened, mutations were detected only in one and three nevi, respectively. In one individual, both nevi screened did not show mutations either in *B-RAF* or *N-RAS* (Table 5 in "Materials and Methods"). Gene expression profiles of eighteen melanocytic nevi harbouring the V600E mutation in the *B-RAF* gene were analysed and compared with expression profiles of four melanocytic nevi without mutations in the *B-RAF* and *N-RAS* genes. Additionally, expression data of melanocytic nevi with or without V600E *B-RAF* mutation were compared with expression profiles of nine non-nevus skin tissues. Microarray data were analysed with GCOS and data were sorted using DMT. Marker analysis was performed using GeneCluster2.0.

Results from microarray data analysed with GCOS

Expression analysis using the GCOS module showed that an average of 51.9% (11 573 ± 450.4) of transcripts were present in the melanocytic nevi harbouring the *B-RAF* mutation, an average of 52.9% (11 796 ± 596.7) of transcripts were present in nevi without this mutation and an average of 51.7% (11 516 ± 505.4) of transcripts were present in non-nevus tissues. From pair-wise comparison of microarray data from nevi harbouring the V600E *B-RAF* mutation with nevi without this mutation 72 data sets were obtained. Similarly, expression profiles of nevi with V600E *B-RAF* mutation were compared with data from non-nevus tissues, yielding 72 data sets. From comparison of nevi without the *B-RAF* mutation with non-nevus tissues 36 data sets were obtained. By comparison of nevi with and without V600E *B-RAF* mutation with non-nevus tissues we obtained 108 data sets. Differentially expressed genes were identified based on the criteria described under "Materials and Methods". In addition, genes scored as significantly "increased" or "decreased" not only in 100%, but also at least 80% in the respective data sets were included in the results.

- *Comparison between melanocytic nevi and non-nevus skin tissues*

209 genes were found to be increased and 138 genes were decreased in melanocytic nevi (with or without the *B-RAF* mutation) when compared to non-nevus skin tissues. Melanocytic nevi of all types show significantly increased expression of known melanocyte markers such as melan-A (*MLANA*, 9-fold), tyrosinase (*TYR*, 13-fold), and dopachrome tautomerase (*DCT*, 5-fold). Other

genes which show distinctive overexpression in melanocytic nevi include endothelin receptor type B (*EDNRB*, 12-fold), ets variant gene 5 (*ETV5*, 10-fold), melanoma antigen family D, 2 and 4 (*MAGED2*, 8-fold, *MAGED4*, 7-fold), melanoma inhibitory activity protein (*MIA*, 8-fold). Tissue inhibitor of metalloproteinase (*TIMP2*) shows 5-fold upregulation, v-akt murine thymoma viral oncogene homolog 3 (*AKT3*) 7-fold, and SRY (sex determining region Y)-box 10 (*SOX10*) is 10-fold upregulated in all melanocytic nevi.

Genes that showed significantly decreased expression in melanocytic nevi include those involved in apoptosis like CASP8 and FADD-like apoptosis regulator (*CFLAR*, 21-fold) and BCL2/adenovirus E1B 19kDa interacting protein 3-like (*BNIP3L*, 5-fold), CD24 antigen (*CD24*, 5-fold), dual specificity phosphatase 5 (*DUSP5*, 10-fold), early growth response 3 (*EGR3*, 6-fold), and tyrosine 3-monooxygenase/tryptophan 5-monooxygenase activation protein (*YWHAZ*, 4-fold). G1 to S phase transition 1 (*GSPT1*), which is involved in the G1/S transition of the mitotic cell cycle, is 8-fold downregulated in melanocytic nevi. Thrombospondin (*THBS1*), which is involved in cell adhesion, shows 8-fold downregulation and inhibitor of DNA binding 1 (*ID1*) 16-fold. Expression of serine proteinase inhibitors, members 13, 3, 4 (*SERPINB13/3/4*) is 8-fold, 5-fold and 17-fold decreased.

• *Identification of differentially expressed genes in melanocytic nevi with V600E B-RAF mutation*
In order to see the effect of the V600E substitution in *B-RAF* on global gene expression we compared the microarray data from melanocytic nevi with and without such mutations. We found 93 genes were significantly upregulated and 104 genes downregulated in nevi with the mutation (Appendix, Tables 14 and 15).

Among the genes prominently upregulated in nevi with the V600E *B-RAF* mutation were those involved in cell adhesion, such as cadherin 19, type 2 (*CDH19*, 23-fold), cell adhesion molecule with homology to L1CAM (*CHL1*, 9-fold), and CD44 antigen (*CD44*, 3-fold). Various upregulated genes, such as fibroblast growth factor 2 (*FGF2*, 6-fold), dual specificity phosphatase 6 (*DUSP6*, 4-fold), cyclin G1 (*CCNG1*, 3-fold), and cyclin I (*CCNI*, 4-fold) function in cell cycle regulation. The tumour suppressor genes cyclin-dependend kinase inhibitor 1C and 2A (*CDKN1C, CDKN2A*) were upregulated 5-fold and 6-fold, respectively in nevi with the mutation. Other genes with increased expression included sprouty homolog 2 (Drosophila, *SPRY2*, 3-fold), S-phase kinase-associated protein 1A (*SKP1A*, 4-fold), microphtalmia-associated transcription factor (*MITF*, 4-fold), G protein-coupled receptor 37 (*GPR37*, 11-fold), nuclear receptor subfamily 3, group C, member 1 (*NR3C1*, 4-fold), pleiotropin (*PTN*, 10-fold), ets variant gene 1 (*ETV1*, 12-fold), and tyrosine 3-

monooxygenase/tryptophan 5-monooxygenase activation protein (*YWHAE*, 6-fold) (Appendix, Table 14).

Matrix metalloproteinase 28 (*MMP28*, 8-fold), cyclin-dependend kinase (CDC2-like) 10 (*CDK10*, 6-fold), FOS-like antigen 2 (*FOSL2*, 6-fold), macrophage stimulating 1 receptor (*MST1R*, 4-fold), and wingless-type MMTV integration site family, member 4 (*WNT4*, 4-fold) were downregulated in melanocytic nevi harbouring the V600E mutation. P53-regulated apoptosis-inducing protein 1 (*P53AIP1*, 9-fold) and necrosis factor receptor superfamily, member 25 (*TNFRSF25*, 4-fold) were other downregulated genes, which also included growth arrest-specific 6 (*GAS6*, 4-fold) that functions in cell growth regulation. Genes of the Ras signalling cascade, such as v-Ha-ras Harvey rat sarcoma viral oncogene homolog (*HRAS*), related RAS viral (r-ras) oncogene homolog (*RRAS*), and Ras interacting protein 1 (*RASIP1*) also showed downregulation (Appendix, Table 15).

• *Differentially expressed genes common to melanoma cell lines and melanocytic nevi with V600E B-RAF mutation*

A comparison of upregulated genes in melanoma cell lines (see 4.4.) and melanocytic nevi showed an overlap of 10 upregulated genes and 5 downregulated genes (Table 16).

Table 16. Genes up- and downregulated in both nevi and melanoma cell lines with V600E mutation.

Gene name	Fold Change	
	Melanocytic nevi	Melanoma cell lines
Upregulated		
• dual specificity phosphatase 6 (*DUSP6*)	3.6	13
• sprouty homolog 2 (*SPRY2*)	3.1	15
• ets variant gene 1 (*ETV1*)	12.0	217
• protein phosphatase 1 (*PPP1R3C*)	4.6	10
• KIAA0470	11.7	11
• paternally expressed 10 (*PEG10*)	9.0	126
• S100 calcium binding protein, beta, (neural) (*S100B*)	6.9	439
• sarcoglycan, epsilon (*SGCE*)	5.7	90
• serine (or cysteine) proteinase inhibitor, clade E (*SERPINE2*)	7.7	6
• solute carrier family 16 (monocarboxylic acid transporter), member 4 (*SLC16A4*)	8.1	227
Downregulated		
• tropomyosin 2 (beta) (*TPM2*)	13.4	14
• macrophage stimulating 1 receptor (*MST1R*)	3.7	7
• jagged 2 (*JAG2*)	5.2	22
• sodium channel, nonvoltage-gated 1 alpha (*SCNN1A*)	2.7	28
• sema domain, immunoglobulin domain (Ig), short basic domain, secreted (semaphorin) 3F (*SEMA3F*)	3.6	4

Results from microarray data analysed with GeneCluster2.0

For analysis of the microarray data using GeneCluster2.0 filter criteria as described in "Materials and Methods" were used. When the expression data of 31 microarrays (9 non-nevus tissues, 4 nevi without and 18 nevi with V600E *B-RAF* mutation) were analysed, 6222 probe sets passed these criteria.

In the first analysis two groups were defined; non-nevus tissues and melanocytic nevi. Supervised analysis of the data demonstrate a clear separation of the non-nevus tissues from the group of melanocytic nevi, whether or not they harbour the V600E mutation in the *B-RAF* gene. Figure 18 shows a selection of 50 best correlated markers which were distinct for each of the two sample groups. Differential expression of a number of genes, which include typical melanocyte markers, clearly distinguish normal skin and melanocytic nevi and support the results obtained from GCOS.

The second analysis was performed with nevi with and without the V600E *B-RAF* mutation as separate groups. Expression data of the two groups of nevi were compared with normal skin tissues. Figure 19 displays a set of 30 best correlated markers that separate the 3 groups of samples. Non-nevus tissues, nevi with and without *B-RAF* mutation were clearly separated by differential expression of a set of genes.

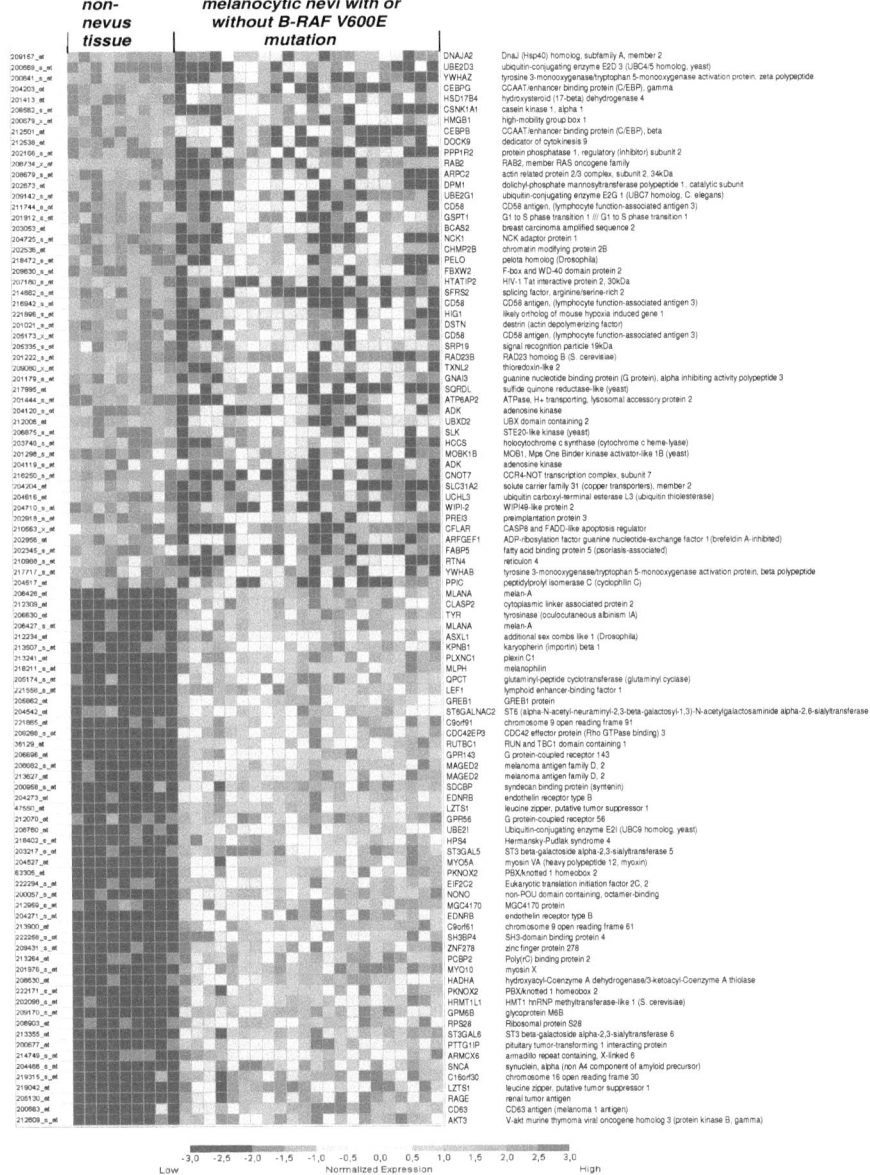

Figure 18. Marker gene analysis showing 50 best correlated genes with differential expression in melanocytic nevi with or without V600E *B-RAF* mutation and normal skin tissue. Markers were selected by computing the Signal to Noise score. The columns shown represent individual samples and rows represent single genes and are ranked in a `best-correlated` order. The colour scale identifies relative gene expression changes normalised by the standard deviation, with 0 representing the mean expression level of a given gene across the panel.

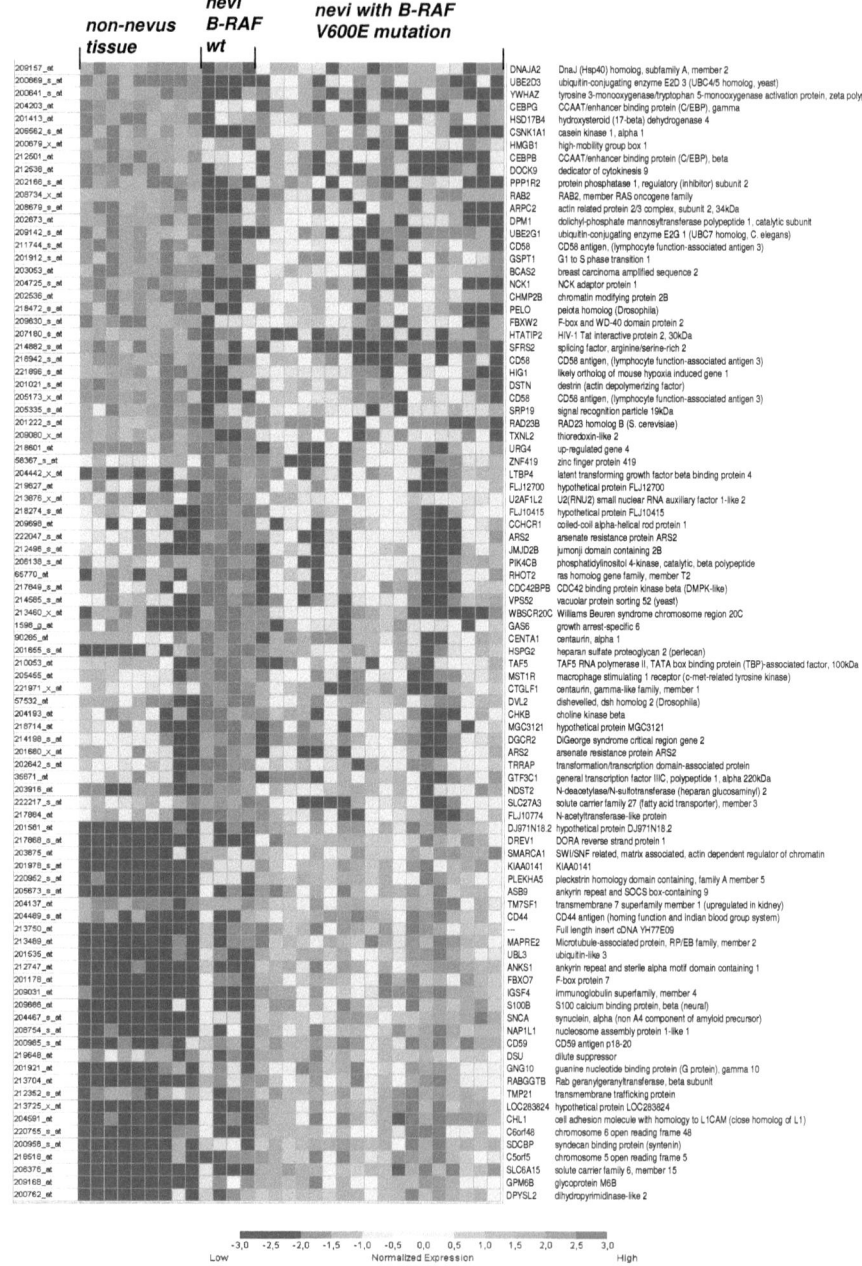

Figure 19. Results from a marker gene analysis of microarray data with 30 best correlated genes in melanocytic nevi with V600E *B-RAF* mutation, nevi without such mutation, and normal skin tissue.

Results of gene ontology analysis using the Gene Ontology Mining Tool (Affymetrix)
In order to obtain a statistical estimate about the over-representation of genes related to a specific biological process, microarray data were applied to the Gene Ontology Mining Tool (Affymetrix). Application of the list of the 93 upregulated genes in nevi with V600E mutation to the Gene Ontology Mining Tool showed over-representation of proportionally various genes in cellular metabolism (36 genes). A high proportion of those genes (15 genes) play roles in protein metabolism, including protein modification, -folding, -biosynthesis, and -catabolism. Such genes included dual specificity phosphatase 6 (*DUSP6*), nucleophosmin/nucleoplasmin 3 (*NPM3*), and heat shock 70kDa protein 8 (*HSPA8*). 13 out of the 36 genes function in nucleobase, nucleoside, nucleotide and nucleic acid metabolism, which included ets variant gene 1 (*ETV1*), microphthalmia-associated transcription factor (*MITF*), and nuclear receptor subfamily 3, member 1 (*NR3C1*).

Likewise, 105 genes were found significantly downregulated in melanocytic nevi with V600E B-RAF mutation. Most of those genes mapped to physiological processes (68 genes) and/or cell communication processes (43 genes). Out of the 68 genes involved in physiological processes, 18 genes played roles in transport processes. V-Ha-ras Harvey rat sarcoma viral oncogene homolog (*HRAS*), related Ras viral (r-ras)oncogene homolog (*RRAS*), or collagen type VI, alpha 2 (*COL6A2*) were examples of such genes. 12 genes functioned in nucleobase, nucleoside, nucleotide and nucleic acid metabolism, such as FOS-like antigen 2 (*FOSL2*), endothelial cell growth factor 1 (*ECGF1*), or ubiquitin-activating enzyme E1 (*UBE1*). 43 genes mapped to cell communication processes, which included 10 that played a role in cell adhesion and 34 genes in signal transduction. Genes with functions in cell adhesion included integrin, beta 4 (*ITGB4*), laminin, alpha 5 (*LAMA5*), and protocadherin 21 (*PCDH21*). Of the 34 genes that mapped to signal transduction, 9 belonged to the sub-group of G-protein-coupled receptor signalling pathways, which included leukotriene B4 receptor (*LTB4R*) and Rap guanine nucleotide exchange factor (GEF)-like 1 (*RAPGEFL1*).

5. DISCUSSION

5.1. Mutations in the B-RAF and N-RAS genes and alterations of the CDKN2A gene locus in melanoma cell lines

We found a high frequency of mutual exclusive mutations in *B-RAF* and *N-RAS* genes mutations in our series of melanoma cell lines. Out of 106 of the investigated individuals, 58 (55%) carried *B-RAF* mutations and 29 (27%) mutations in *N-RAS*. The distribution of mutations in those genes in melanoma is in good agreement with previous reports (193, 197-199, 218). The predominant mutation which we detected in the *B-RAF* gene was a single base substitution in the kinase activation domain involving codon 600 that has been described before (193, 198). The V600E mutant probably mimics the activational phosphorylation of the adjacent residue (193, 198). This residue is identical at the corresponding positions in *C-RAF* and *A-RAF*, and is conserved through the evolution with a single exception of *Drosophila Raf* homologue (193, 243). The mutant V600E has been reported to possess a high basal activity, and it induces focus formation in NIH3T3 cells with much higher efficiency than the wild-type BRAF (193). Though mutations in *B-RAF* are of common occurrence in melanoma, the distribution varies according to tumour location. In addition to V600E, in five individuals a valine-to-lysine change at codon 600 (V600K) through GT1798-1799AA tandem mutation was detected. The detection of valine-to-lysine changes confirms the possibility of B-RAF activation through substitution with both positively and negatively charged amino acids (200, 244). The most frequent *N-RAS* mutations in our study occured in codon 61, which is in agreement with results from other studies (197, 218).

The mutual exclusiveness of *B-RAF* and *N-RAS* mutations in our melanoma cell lines indicates that the activation of RAS or B-RAF leads to the same phenotype in melanomas and other cancers (200, 245). In our studies we found a high frequency of mutual exclusive mutations in *B-RAF* and *N-RAS* genes also in benign melanocytic nevi, which are putative precursor lesions of melanoma. This observation together with other reports underlines the centrality of B-RAF/N-RAS in melanoma biology and provides further evidence that such mutations occur early in melanocyte transformation and persist through melanoma progression (200, 202, 219). The fact that not all melanocytic nevi harbouring *B-RAF* or *N-RAS* mutations progress to melanoma leads to the hypothesis that activated N-RAS or B-RAF alone is not able to transform human melanocytes, but require additional cooperating events for tumour formation.

Besides *B-RAF* and *N-RAS* mutations, we found a high frequency of homozygous deletions of the *CDKN2A* locus genes in our melanoma cell lines. Deletion of the *CDKN2A* gene locus has been detected in ~50% of primary melanomas and nearly all melanoma cell lines (124, 125). Interestingly, in a high percentage of the individuals investigated in our study, we found an overlap of *B-RAF* or *N-RAS* mutations and *CDKN2A* deletions. However, no deletion or mutation in *CDKN2A* in melanocytic nevi have been reported (246, 247). These data together with our observations in metastatic melanoma cell lines indicate that *CDKN2A* deletions are not early events in melanomagenesis but arise in later stage in melanocyte transformation. In a recent study it was shown that sustained V600E *B-RAF* expression in human melanocytes results in cell cycle arrest, accompanied by the induction of both p16 and senescence-associated acidic beta-galactosidase (SA-beta-Gal) activity (42). This finding indicated that melanocytic nevi undergo *B-RAF* V600E-induced senescence and p16 contributes to the protection against *B-RAF* V600E-driven cell proliferation. Our data show that *CDKN2A* alterations in melanoma overlap with *B-RAF/N-RAS* mutations. Thus, we hypothesise that loss of the tumour suppressor *CDKN2A* with resulting loss of p16 function constitutes a second genetic event, in addition to activating mutations in *B-RAF* or *N-RAS*, in melanocytes to overcome senescence and to undergo malignant transformation. These genetic events occur in different stages of melanocyte transformation and appear to be preserved during melanoma progression up to the metastatic stage. Further, our data also point to a cooperative role of RAS-RAF-MEK-ERK and Rb pathways in melanoma formation. However, 16% of the patients in our study carried no mutations in the investigated genes, indicating that alterations in genes other than *B-RAF*, *N-RAS* or *CDKN2A* could also be involved in melanomagenesis which merit further investigation.

Besides a high number of melanocytic nevi, epidemiologic data support a role of UV exposure with increased melanoma risk (110, 248). However, the mechanism involved for the role of exposure to UV light is complex. Though, in rare instances UV signature mutations in melanoma have been reported (146). The incidence of melanoma appears to be higher in populations who develop melanocytic nevi early in life, and evidently increased sun exposure is related to the number of nevi (249). However, *B-RAF* mutations are common in melanomas arising in areas intermittently exposed to the sun, but are rare in melanomas on skin that is chronically exposed to the sun or on acral skin and mucosal membranes that are seldom or never exposed to the sun (250). It has been suggested that UV radiation plays a role in the genesis of *N-RAS* mutations in melanoma (222, 223). The two most frequent mutations that we observed in our series of melanoma cell lines (a CAA to AAA transversion, Q61K; and a CAA to CGA transition, Q61R, respectively) have both been shown to be induced by UV radiation *in vitro* and have also been described at high frequencies for UVB induced lesions (251). Moreover, frequent loss of p16 has been reported in melanomas arising on sun-exposed skin, whereas in melanoma cells from sun-protected skin p16 expression was preserved (252-254). These observations contribute to the suggestion of a molecular link between sunlight exposure and melanoma.

In summary, our data showed a high frequency of *B-RAF* and *N-RAS* mutations and overlapping homozygous deletion of the *CDKN2A* locus genes in melanoma. Thus, our data suggest an overlapping and cooperating role of these genes in melanoma formation.

5.2. Expression of B-RAF, N-RAS and CDKN2A and correlation with mutations in melanoma cell lines

Besides activating mutations, overexpression of B-RAF has been reported to be one of the mechanisms for constitutive activation of the MAPK pathway (242). Similarly, not only oncogenic mutations of K-RAS, but amplification and consequent overexpression of even wild-type K-RAS were shown to contribute to tumour growth (255). However, in melanoma, most of reports show elevated activity mainly through oncogenic mutation (206, 256, 257). Our analysis of B-RAF expression in melanoma cell lines showed a highly significant inverse association with *N-RAS* mutations. Conversely, our data also showed elevated expression of B-RAF in cell lines with *B-RAF* mutation, though the relation was not statistically significant. However, our data are in contrast with an earlier study which showed overexpression of B-RAF protein in melanoma cells that carried wild-type B-RAF and N-RAS (242). In another interesting observation, we found that N-RAS expression was significantly lower in cell lines with *CDKN2A* homozygous deletion and this effect was independent of *B-RAF* and *N-RAS* mutational status. Activation of RAS and other downstream effectors leads to senescence response through induction of p16, however, reduced expression in cell lines with *CDKN2A* deletion is difficult to explain (258). However, we suggest a possibility of a feedback loop mechanism where loss of p16 and ARF could ablate the requirement for RAS activation.

5.3. Absence of the AKAP9-B-RAF fusion transcript in melanoma cell lines

The V600E *B-RAF* mutation is believed to produce a constitutively active kinase by disrupting hydrophobic interactions between residues in the activation loop and residues in the ATP binding site that maintain the inactive conformation, allowing development of new interactions that fold the kinase into a catalytically active structure (195). Correspondingly, V600E B-RAF exhibits elevated basal kinase activity (193). Conceivably, other alterations that would release the inhibitory constrains of the catalytic domain of B-RAF could also result in kinase activation. Loss of the N-terminal regulatory domains as a result of fusion to different genes has been shown to activate B-RAF kinase and transform NIH3T3 cells (259, 260). However, until recently this mechanism of B-RAF activation has not been identified in human tumours. Lately, activation of B-RAF by chromosomal rearrangement resulting in an in-frame fusion between *B-RAF* and *AKAP9* and in its N-terminal truncation has been reported in papillary thyroid carcinomas with history of radiation exposure. *B-RAF* point mutations were absent in those tumours. The fusion gene exhibited elevated basal kinase activity, stimulated ERK phosphorylation, and induced transformation of NIH3T3 cells (212).

To clarify whether such a chromosomal rearrangement resulting in the oncogenic AKAP9 – B-RAF fusion transcript contributes to the activation of the MAPK pathway also in melanoma, we screened our melanoma cell lines for the presence of the fusion gene. We did not detect the AKAP9 – B-RAF fusion transcript in our melanoma cell lines, independently of the presence of *B-RAF* mutations. This finding suggests that paracentric chromosomal inversions represent a common genetic mechanism of radiation-associated carcinogenesis. Moreover, this observation points to a tissue-specificity of the occurrence of this chromosomal rearrangement. Due to our observation that 80% of our melanoma cell lines harboured activating mutations in *B-RAF* and mutually exclusive in *N-RAS* we conclude that those alterations constitute the prevalent genetic mechanism of activation of the MAPK pathway in melanoma.

5.4. Effects of common genetic alterations on gene expression in melanoma cell lines and melanocytic nevi

5.4.1. Effect of B-RAF (V600E) and N-RAS (Q61R) mutations on global gene expression in melanoma cell lines

Though a discernible picture of effects of the B-RAF and N-RAS mutants in melanoma cell lines has begun to emerge, however, the consequences of these mutants on global gene expression remain to be understood. To date only one study based on cDNA microarrays has identified differences in expression between cell lines with and without *B-RAF* and *N-RAS* mutations (241).

In our study we investigated the global gene expression profile of melanoma cell lines with focus on the the most potent and common mutation V600E in the *B-RAF* gene and the common Q61R mutation in the *N-RAS* gene. Our results from stringent analysis of the expression data, from melanoma cell lines with and without mutations, partly validated by quantitative real-time PCR showed (a) upregulation and downregulation of a number of genes with diverse and disparate molecular functions in cell lines with *B-RAF* and *N-RAS* mutations against cell lines without mutations; (b) overlapping sets of over- and underexpressed genes in cell lines with *B-RAF* and *N-RAS* mutations; and (c) distinct sets of up- or downregulated genes that distinguish the cell lines with *B-RAF* and *N-RAS* mutations. Many of the genes with affected expression in melanoma cell lines due to mutations in the *B-RAF* and *N-RAS* genes encode constituents or regulators of the RAS-RAF-MEK-ERK and related pathways or are associated with metastasis or tumour invasiveness.

The group of genes prominently upregulated in melanoma cell lines with mutant *B-RAF* and *N-RAS* with potential direct or indirect role in the MAPK pathways included a dual specificity phosphatase gene, *DUSP6*; an inhibitor of MAPK signalling, *SPRY2*; a 14-3-3 binding protein encoding gene, *TAZ*; and oncogenic *AKT3* (261-264). DUSP6 with a presumptive growth suppressor role causes both induction and inactivation of ERK1/2 through a potential feed back loop mechanism that involves non-catalytic binding (265). The localization of DUSP6 in cytoplasm has been reported to effectively prevent translocation of ERK to target effectors inside the nucleus (261). The overexpression of DUSP6 can be speculated to have a potential analogous role in rescue of hyper-phosphorylated 'inactive' B-RAF (through a feed back loop), though, the putative phosphorylating sites in B-RAF similar to those discovered in C-RAF are not known (266).

Further in concordance with an earlier report, we not only found relative overexpression of SPRY2, an inhibitor of MAPK signalling in cell lines with *B-RAF* mutation, but also in cell lines with mutant *N-RAS*, albeit at lower level than in cell lines with mutant *B-RAF* (267, 268). In cell lines with mutations we also found relative overexpression of AKT3, which has been specifically shown to be deregulated at a high frequency in sporadic melanoma through an increased gene copy number and decreased PTEN expression (264). Interestingly, B-RAF contains several AKT phosphorylation sites and mutations affecting those residues have been reported in lung cancer (198). The inhibitory nature of AKT mediated phosphorylation of B-RAF together with overexpression observed in melanoma cells with mutant *B-RAF* and *N-RAS* highlight the complexities of cellular regulation or deregulation.

Some of the genes with distinct overexpression only in cell lines containing the *B-RAF* mutation included the *FYN* oncogene, genes belonging to melanoma antigen family, mitochondrial folate transporter and matrix metalloproteinase 14 (*MMP14*) (269, 270). Whereas glutathione S-transferase M4 (*GSTM4*) and Ras-related GTP binding D (*RRAGD*) were the genes upregulated specifically in cell lines with the *N-RAS* mutation compared to cell lines without mutations. Other overexpressed transcripts specific for cell lines with the *N-RAS* mutations included ets gene variants, which belong to a family of oncogenic transcription factors, several G-coupled protein receptors and dual specificity phosphatase 4 (265, 271).

Differential expression of melanoma antigen, family A, 3 (*MAGEA3*) and melan-A (*MLANA*), both of which are frequently expressed in melanomas, has been identified as a good discriminator between different groups and stages of melanoma in several studies (272-274). In our study we observed, that upregulation of those two genes was associated with the mutations in *B-RAF* and *N-RAS*, respectively. Interestingly, the tumour antigen *MAGEA3* was significantly associated with the V600E *B-RAF* mutation, whereas upregulation of the major melanocyte differentiation antigen *MLANA* was only seen in cell lines harbouring the Q61R mutation in *N-RAS*. Our data not only confirm the presence of *MAGEA3* and *MLANA* as important markers in melanoma progression, but also point to a mutation-specific gene regulation of these two genes.

In cell lines with *B-RAF* and *N-RAS* mutations we found lack of IL-18 cytokine expression, which is identified as a strong inducer of interferon-γ and its constitutive production can lead to an enhanced anti-tumour response and improved survival (275). Other genes with significantly reduced expression in cell lines with *B-RAF* and *N-RAS* mutation included *CD24* antigen, Krüppel-like factors 4 and 5 (*KLF4* and *5*) and inhibitor of DNA-binding 2 (*ID2*) (276-278). CD24, a small heavily glycosylated mucin-like glycosylphosphatidyl-inositol-linked cell surface protein is expressed in a wide variety of human malignancies and is associated with a potential to metastasise (276). Notably, the loss of expression of some of the genes was more pronounced in cell lines with *B-RAF* mutation than in cell lines with *N-RAS* mutation.

Interestingly, we found twice as many upregulated genes in cell lines carrying *N-RAS* mutations than in those carrying mutations in *B-RAF*, with an overlap of only 9%. This difference in the influence on the global gene expression could be the putative influence on prognosis of the patients with different mutations in tumours. Evidently, pathway analysis of the affected genes suggested that the V600E mutation in *B-RAF* mainly affects the ERK signalling pathway, whereas the Q61R *N-RAS* mutation mainly causes perturbation of expression of genes involved in the PI3K/AKT apoptotic pathway (data not shown). Indeed, this finding is in good agreement with a recent report, where suppression of oncogenic N-RAS harbouring the Q61R mutation resulted in decreased phosphorylation of AKT and increased apoptosis (224). The hypothesis of melanoma development via distinct genetic pathways involving *B-RAF* and *N-RAS* mutations, has been earlier discussed (279). Our data support the hypothesis that mutated N-RAS activates both the PI3K/AKT and MAPK pathways, whereas mutated B-RAF seems to activate only the latter.

Our results provide novel insight into the effect of mutations in the *B-RAF* and *N-RAS* genes on global gene expression in melanoma and highlight the complexity of mechanisms involved in tumour initiation and maintenance. In melanoma cell lines, we have shown the effect of the V600E mutation in *B-RAF* and the Q61R mutation in *N-RAS* on the transcription of various genes, many of which are involved in RAS/RAF-signalling and related pathways. The extent to which these results can be reproduced *in situ* remains to be seen. Moreover, gene expression analysis alone cannot provide an overall integrative molecular understanding of the genesis of melanoma. Our findings provide a good basis for further evaluation through functional studies. In further sense the data presented here may prove to encode useful new therapeutic targets, involving both MAPK and PI3K/AKT pathways, to efficiently treat patients with melanomas carrying the V600E *B-RAF* or the Q61R *N-RAS* mutations.

5.4.2. Effect of homozygous deletion of the CDKN2A locus genes on global gene expression in melanoma cell lines

The *CDKN2A* locus on chromosome 9p21 in an unusual genomic organization encodes two unrelated tumour suppressors and is regularly inactivated in a variety of human cancers (146). Besides mutations, the *CDKN2A* locus genes are frequent targets for homozygous deletions in tumours or are silenced through *de novo* promoter hypermethylation. Homozygous deletion of the *CDKN2A* locus, including the homologous *CDKN2B* gene, results in growth advantage to tumour cells due to simultaneous loss of more than one tumour suppressor. However, based on micro-deletion pattern in a subset of tumours, it is argued to be a specific mechanism of ARF inactivation. This argument is supported by (a) unlike p16, mutations in tumours exclusive to ARF transcripts are enigmatically rare; (b) involvement of multiple rather than specific domains in its binding to MDM2; and (c) instances of specific deletion, both somatic and germline, of exon 1β (115, 119, 280). However the frequency of homozygous deletions in tumours tend to remain underestimated as contaminating stromal cells limit the efficiency of PCR based techniques and paucity of DNA from tumour samples, preclude the use of robust techniques like Southern hybridization (115, 281). Therefore within obvious limitations, homogeneity of tumour cell lines provides an advantage for the detection of homozygous deletions and for studying consequent effects. Besides activating mutations in *B-RAF* and *N-RAS* proto-oncogenes, homozygous deletion of the *CDKN2A* gene is suspected to generate a second major genetic event promoting melanocyte transformation into melanoma.

To investigate the molecular consequences of the homozygous deletion of the *CDKN2A* locus genes, we compared the global gene expression in melanoma cell lines with and without such deletions. In order to avoid complexities, we confirmed that the selected cell lines did not carry mutations in the *B-RAF* and *N-RAS* genes. Homozygous deletions were reliably detected by quantitative real-time PCR and the cell lines without deletion expressed CDKN2A. We found a large heterogeneity in genes up- and downregulated in cell lines with deletion. Stringent analysis of microarray data showed differential expression of genes involved in various cellular functions that included structural, transporter, transcription, binding, signal transduction and other activities.

Pathway analysis showed that out of 156 differentially expressed genes in cell lines with *CDKN2A* deletion, 112 mapped to known pathways and functions. 43 genes were involved in cell death and cell invasion (data not shown). Genes with differential regulation included secreted protein acidic and rich in cysteine (*SPARC,* 128-fold upregulation), which is a matrix-associated protein that elicits changes in cell shape, inhibits cell cycle progression, and influences the synthesis of extracellular matrix genes. Dopachrome tautomerase (*DCT*, 46-fold upregulation) and tyrosinase (*TYR*, 66-fold upregulation) are melanocyte-specific genes that are involved in regulation of melanin synthesis (282). Importantly, dopachrome tautomerase has been reported to be activated by microphthalmia-associated transcription factor MITF (283). MITF also activates p16 expression, inducing cell cycle arrest (284). Overexpression of DCT in melanoma cell lines with *CDKN2A* deletion could probably reflect amplification of *MITF* in these cell lines. Earlier, *MITF* in its oncogenic role has been shown to be amplified in metastatic melanoma with *B-RAF* mutation and p16 inactivation (225).

Integrin, beta 3 (*ITGB3*, 33-fold upregulation) belongs to the family of integrins, which are known to participate in cell adhesion as well as cell-surface mediated signalling. S-phase kinase-associated protein 2 (*SKP2*, 7-fold downregulation) encodes a member of the F-box protein family. Interestingly, SKP2 has been suggested to be essential for S-phase entry of the cell cycle (285). Inhibitors of DNA binding 1 and 2 (*ID1*, 27-fold downregulation; *ID2*, 3-fold downregulation) play a role in the negative regulation of cell differentiation. *ID1* and *ID2* both belong to the same gene family and exert their molecular effects through the same mechanism. However, downregulation of *ID1* was more than *ID2*. ID1 has been shown to interact directly with p16, while no such evidence has been shown for ID2 (286).

Earlier we had detected specific upregulation of *MAGEA3* in cell lines with the *B-RAF* mutation. However, in the present study we found over 90-, 120- and 600-fold upregulation of *MAGEA2*, *A6* and *A12*, respectively in cell lines with homozygous deletion of the *CDKN2A* gene. *MAGEA* genes encode a group of cancer/testis antigens that are recognized by autologous cytolytic T-lymphocytes in association with HLA molecules. *MAGEA* genes because of repressed promoter methylation are expressed in a variety of malignant tissues and with the exception of testis and placenta are absent in normal tissues. The products of these genes have been considered as targets for active immunotherapy (287, 288). One of the limitations associated with immune therapy is expression of tumour specific antigens. Therefore, the high levels of expression of specific melanoma antigens in melanoma cell lines with homozygous deletion of the *CDKN2A* gene, if confirmed in a large number of cell lines and tumour tissues, could be useful in identification of a subset of melanoma patients for therapeutic considerations (289).

Surprisingly, we found an overlap of differential expression of several genes in the cell lines with homozygous deletion of the *CDKN2A* gene and in cell lines with mutations in the *B-RAF* and *N-RAS* genes (and intact *CDKN2A* locus). Cluster analysis of our microarray data revealed a subset of genes that separated melanoma cell lines with mutations in the *B-RAF/N-RAS* genes or homozygous deletion of the *CDKN2A* locus from the cell lines without such alterations. Again, confirmed by our and other studies, most of the melanoma cell lines (and melanoma tissues) carry mutations in *B-RAF/N-RAS* genes and alterations in the *CDKN2A* locus simultaneously. However, it is possible that the small number of melanomas without alterations in any of these genes constitute a subgroup with a different gene regulation pattern with possible therapeutic consequences. Some of the genes upregulated in cell lines with homozygous deletion of *CDKN2A* locus and also in cell lines with *B-RAF* or *N-RAS* mutations included dual specificity phosphatases 4 and 6; *SPRY2*, which is an inhibitor of MAP-kinase signaling; *TAZ*, a 14-3-3 binding protein; and oncogenic *AKT3* (261-264). The relative overexpression of several genes that encode constituents or regulators of the RAS-RAF-MEK-ERK pathway, in the cell lines with the *CDKN2A* deletion and likewise in the cell lines with *B-RAF* or *N-RAS* mutations, highlights the ubiquitous role of this pathway in tumour initiation, maintenance and invasion. The commonly downregulated genes in melanoma cell lines with homozygous deletion of the *CDKN2A* gene and cell lines with *B-RAF/N-RAS* mutations included interleukin 18 (*IL18*), inhibitor of DNA binding 2 (*ID2*), Krüppel like factors 4 and 5 (*KLF4* and *5*), and *CD24* antigen (276, 278). Again, we observed a deregulation of several genes that encode constituents or regulators of the RAS-RAF-MEK-ERK pathway and genes involved in cell cycle regulation, some of which were up- or downregulated both in the cell lines with the *CDKN2A* deletion and independently in the cell lines with *B-RAF* or *N-RAS* mutations. This finding leads to the speculation, that the overall effects of gene deregulation might add up in melanomas harbouring both those genetic events.

Altogether, our data from comparative microarray analysis showed a differential regulation of several classes of genes involved in different functional regulatory pathways in cell lines with and without homozygous deletion of the *CDKN2A* gene. Our results suggest that the study of differential expression patterns due to genetic alterations at a single locus can provide an insight into molecular mechanisms from identification of specifically affected pathways. Overexpression of specific melanoma antigens in cell lines with homozygous deletion merits further study and *in situ* confirmation, as it can potentially influence the treatment in a sub-set of melanoma.

5.4.3. Effect of the V600E B-RAF mutation on global gene expression in melanocytic nevi

The high frequency of *B-RAF* mutations in benign melanocytiv nevi, with the V600E exchange being most prominent, suggests that these alterations constitute a crucial step in melanoma initiation (200, 202). In earlier studies gene expression profiles comparing melanocytic nevi and different stages of melanoma have been carried out (238, 290). However, no study has been performed to explore the changes of gene expression due to the V600E *B-RAF* mutation in the early stages of melanocyte transformation. In a step forward from earlier studies we also used microarray technology to define differences in gene expression profiles of melanocytic nevi with and without the oncogenic V600E *B-RAF* mutation. We also compared expression profiles from nevi with those from normal skin tissues. Moreover, we compared the data obtained from nevi with data from our previous study performed on melanoma cell lines. We also have attempted to hypothesize the links between the occurrence of V600E mutation of the *B-RAF* gene, resulting gene expression patterns and the possible role in melanoma initiation.

Stringent analysis of microarray data a) confirmed known differences in gene expression between melanocytic nevi and normal skin, b) showed significant differences in gene expression of nevi with and without the V600E *B-RAF* mutation, c) also showed a number of genes expressed differentially in nevi with mutation overlapped with those observed in melanoma cell lines with similar mutation. Out of 14 500 genes on the the HG-U133A2.0 microarray, 209 were upregulated and 138 downregulated in melanocytic compared to non-nevus skin tissue. Overexpressed genes in melanocytic nevi of all types included known melanocyte markers such as melan-A (*MLANA*), tyrosinase (*TYR*), and dopachrome tautomerase (*DCT*). Other genes which show distinctive overexpression in melanocytic nevi include endothelin receptor type B (*EDNRB*), melanoma antigen family D, 2 and 4 (*MAGED2, MAGED4*), melanoma inhibitory activity protein (*MIA*), tissue inhibitor of metalloproteinase (*TIMP2*), and v-akt murine thymoma viral oncogene homolog 3 (*AKT3*). Genes with significantly decreased expression in melanocytic nevi included genes involved in apoptosis like CASP8 and FADD-like apoptosis regulator (*CFLAR*) and BCL2/adenovirus E1B 19kDa interacting protein 3-like (*BNIP3L*); genes regulating G1-S phase transition of the cell cycle, G1 to S phase transition 1 (*GSPT1*) and inhibitor of DNA binding 1 (*ID1*); a member of dual specificity phosphatases, dual specificity phosphatase 5 (*DUSP5*); and UV-repressible serine (or cysteine) proteinase inhibitor, members 13 (*SERPINB13*).

In melanocytic nevi with V600E *B-RAF* mutation, 93 genes were upregulated and 105 downregulated compared to nevi without mutation. Interestingly, we found the tumour suppressors cyclin-dependend kinase inhibitors 1C and 2A (*CDKN1C, CDKN2A*) significantly upregulated in melanocytic nevi with *B-RAF* mutation. In an earlier study it has been shown that sustained V600E *B-RAF* expression in human melanocytes leads to cell cycle arrest, accompanied by the induction of p16 and senescence-associated acidic beta-galactosidase activity (42). In concordance with that observation, the data presented here indicate that in melanocytic nevi V600E *B-RAF* oncogenic activation leads to CDKN2A overexpression, suggesting that CDKN2A functions as an essential mediator of oncogene-induced senescence preventing progression to melanoma.

Several studies linked increased expression of fibroblast growth factor 2 (*FGF2*) to the stimulation of angiogenesis and melanoma progression (291, 292). FGF2 expression allows nevus cells to survive and proliferate in the dermis (293). The increased FGF2 expression level which we observed in nevi with V600E *B-RAF* mutation might indicate that oncogenic *B-RAF* activation triggers FGF2 expression and therefore survival and proliferation of nevus cells. The major melanocyte differentiation factor microphthalmia-associated transcription factor (*MITF*) was significantly upregulated in melanocytic nevi with V600E *B-RAF* mutation. Both the V600E *B-RAF* mutation and CDKN2A inactivation have been found to accompany amplification of the *MITF* in melanoma cell lines, suggesting an oncogenic role for MITF (225). In contrast, in melanocytes MITF has been shown to induce CDKN2A expression leading to cell cycle arrest (284). Accordingly, in our experiments on melanocytic nevi we observe overexpression of both MITF and CDKN2A. Moreover, with oncogene-induced activation, MITF seems to function rather as a tumour suppressor than an oncogene, through induction of CDKN2A.

Other prominently upregulated genes in melanocytic nevi with mutations include those involved in cell adhesion, such as cadherin 19, type 2 (*CDH19*) and cell adhesion molecule with homology to L1CAM (*CHL1*); and a member of G-protein coupled receptors, glutamate receptor, ionotropic, AMPA1 (*GRIA1*). Stimulation of oncogenic metabotropic glutamate receptor 1 (*GRM1*) in melanoma cells has been shown to activate ERK1/2 via protein kinase C in absence of *B-RAF* mutations (294). Results from transgenic mouse models provided further evidence for the involvement of glutamate receptors in melanocytic neoplasia (295). Our results further support a fundamental role for glutamate receptors in melanocyte transformation, however, with a strong link to the oncogenic V600E *B-RAF* mutation. The importance of glutamate antagonists as a new promising class of drugs that can contribute significantly to the therapeutic management of different kinds of cancer has been mentioned before (296). A number of genes involved in apoptosis show significant downregulation in melanocytic nevi with V600E *B-RAF* mutation. P53-regulated apoptosis-inducing protein 1 (*P53AIP1*) plays an important role in mediating p53-dependend apoptosis (297). Expression of tumour necrosis factor receptor superfamily, member 25 (*TNFRSF25*) triggers apoptosis in mammalian cells (298). Jagged 2 (*JAG2*) was upregulated in invasive clones from melanoma cell lines (299). However, in our study performed on melanocytic nevi we observed significant downregulation of *JAG2* in nevi with *B-RAF* mutation. JAG2 is a protein originally identified in *Drosophila* cell fate determination as a ligand for members of the Notch gene family (300, 301). The Notch signalling pathway is an evolutionary conserved pathway for local cell-cell communication between neighboring cells (302). Activation of the jagged 2/notch 1 signalling pathway is known to overcome density-dependend inhibition of cell division in confluent fibroblasts (303). Thus, we conclude that downregulation of *JAG2* in melanocytic nevi with activating V600E mutation might comprise an antagonistic mechanism to the sustained MAPK pathway activation mediated by mutated B-RAF.

Genes differentially expressed in both nevi and melanoma cell lines with V600E *B-RAF* mutation included dual specificity phosphatase 6 (*DUSP6*) and sprouty homolog 2 (*SPRY2*). Both genes are inhibitors of MAPK signalling and have been discussed in earlier sections of this thesis. Our data confirm, that activation of the MAPK pathway is an early event in melanomagenesis and is maintained through melanoma progression. Commonly downregulated genes in nevi and melanoma cell lines with V600E *B-RAF* mutation include Jagged 2 (*JAG2*), tropomyosin 2 (*TPM2*) and macrophage stimulating 1 receptor (*MST1R*).

Our data provide novel insight into the effect of the most common and potent V600E mutation in the *B-RAF* gene on global gene expression in melanocytic nevi, putative precursors of malignant melanoma. Our results support the hypothesis that activation of the RAS-RAF-MEK-ERK pathway occurs early, in melanocytic nevi, and is further enhanced with the occurrence of the V600E *B-RAF* mutation. Several tumour suppressing mechanisms antagonise sustained MAPK pathway activation mediated by mutated B-RAF in the early stages of melanocyte transformation. Besides provision of important information increasing the understanding of the molecular mechanisms of melanocyte transformation, the data presented may prove to encode useful new markers for early recognition of individuals with increased risk for development of malignant melanoma.

6. SUMMARY

The overall aim of this study was to understand molecular genetic events and their consequences in cutaneous malignant melanoma. This thesis has focused on the characterisation of somatic alterations in the *B-RAF* and *N-RAS* proto-oncogenes and the tumour suppressor gene *CDKN2A*. We evaluated the consequences of the most prominent mutation in *B-RAF*, V600E; a common mutation in *N-RAS*, Q61R; and homozygous deletion of the *CDKN2A* locus genes on global gene expression in melanoma cell lines. Additionally, we examined the effect of the V600E *B-RAF* mutation on global gene expression in benign melanocytic nevi. The studies were performed on a large series of metastatic melanoma cell lines and benign melanocytic nevi.

Our main findings suggest (a) high frequency of mutually exclusive mutations in *B-RAF* and *N-RAS* genes in melanoma, (b) overlap between mutations in *B-RAF/N-RAS* genes and *CDKN2A* alterations and (c) relationship between expression and alterations of these genes. The data from global gene expression suggest that alterations in *B-RAF*, *N-RAS* and *CDKN2A* in melanoma result in up- and downregulation of several genes involved in critical cellular functions. Similarly, we also detected up- and downregulation of critical genes in melanocytic nevi when compared with non-nevus skin tissue as well as in nevi with *B-RAF* mutation compared to nevi without mutation. Surprisingly, a number of genes upregulated and downregulated were common to both melanoma cell lines and melanocytic nevi with V600E *B-RAF* mutation.

Thus, our results suggest, mutations in the *B-RAF* gene and to a certain extent in *N-RAS* are early but insufficient events that occur in nevi. The loss of *CDKN2A* most likely constitutes a second genetic ʻhitʼ required for melanoma progression. Our data in this study are in accordance with recent findings where escape from initial senescence response due to oncogenic mutation has been shown to require loss of additional check points like p16 and ARF. Further, these alterations cause differential regulation of genes involved in critical cell regulation pathways. Upon further validation these results can be used for identification of molecular targets for prognostic and therapeutic purposes.

7. REFERENCES

1. Hurst, E.A., Harbour, J.W. and Cornelius, L.A. (2003) Ocular melanoma: a review and the relationship to cutaneous melanoma. *Arch Dermatol,* **139,** 1067-73.
2. Lens, M.B. and Dawes, M. (2004) Global perspectives of contemporary epidemiological trends of cutaneous malignant melanoma. *Br J Dermatol,* **150,** 179-85.
3. Martin, R.C. and Robinson, E. (2004) Cutaneous melanoma in Caucasian New Zealanders: 1995-1999. *ANZ J Surg,* **74,** 233-7.
4. MacKie, R.M., Bray, C.A., Hole, D.J., Morris, A., Nicolson, M., Evans, A., Doherty, V. and Vestey, J. (2002) Incidence of and survival from malignant melanoma in Scotland: an epidemiological study. *Lancet,* **360,** 587-91.
5. Diepgen, T.L. and Mahler, V. (2002) The epidemiology of skin cancer. *Br J Dermatol,* **146 Suppl 61,** 1-6.
6. Bevona, C. and Sober, A.J. (2002) Melanoma incidence trends. *Dermatol Clin,* **20,** 589-95, vii.
7. Garbe, C., McLeod, G.R. and Buettner, P.G. (2000) Time trends of cutaneous melanoma in Queensland, Australia and Central Europe. *Cancer,* **89,** 1269-78.
8. Jones, W.O., Harman, C.R., Ng, A.K. and Shaw, J.H. (1999) Incidence of malignant melanoma in Auckland, New Zealand: highest rates in the world. *World J Surg,* **23,** 732-5.
9. Jemal, A., Devesa, S.S., Hartge, P. and Tucker, M.A. (2001) Recent trends in cutaneous melanoma incidence among whites in the United States. *J Natl Cancer Inst,* **93,** 678-83.
10. Bulliard, J.L., Cox, B. and Semenciw, R. (1999) Trends by anatomic site in the incidence of cutaneous malignant melanoma in Canada, 1969-93. *Cancer Causes Control,* **10,** 407-16.
11. Garbe, C. and Blum, A. (2001) Epidemiology of cutaneous melanoma in Germany and worldwide. *Skin Pharmacol Appl Skin Physiol,* **14,** 280-90.
12. Mansson-Brahme, E., Johansson, H., Larsson, O., Rutqvist, L.E. and Ringborg, U. (2002) Trends in incidence of cutaneous malignant melanoma in a Swedish population 1976-1994. *Acta Oncol,* **41,** 138-46.
13. Stracci, F., Minelli, L., D'Alo, D., Fusco-Moffa, I., Falsettini, E., Cassetti, T., Romagnoli, C. and La Rosa, F. (2005) Incidence, mortality and survival trends of cutaneous melanoma in Umbria, Italy. 1978-82 and 1994-98. *Tumori,* **91,** 6-8.
14. Ocana-Riola, R., Martinez-Garcia, C., Serrano, S., Buendia-Eisman, A., Ruiz-Baena, C. and Canela-Soler, J. (2001) Population-based study of cutaneous malignant melanoma in the Granada province (Spain), 1985-1992. *Eur J Epidemiol,* **17,** 169-74.
15. Chen, Y.J., Wu, C.Y., Chen, J.T., Shen, J.L., Chen, C.C. and Wang, H.C. (1999) Clinicopathologic analysis of malignant melanoma in Taiwan. *J Am Acad Dermatol,* **41,** 945-9.
16. Koh, D., Wang, H., Lee, J., Chia, K.S., Lee, H.P. and Goh, C.L. (2003) Basal cell carcinoma, squamous cell carcinoma and melanoma of the skin: analysis of the Singapore Cancer Registry data 1968-97. *Br J Dermatol,* **148,** 1161-6.
17. Hamre, M.R., Chuba, P., Bakhshi, S., Thomas, R. and Severson, R.K. (2002) Cutaneous melanoma in childhood and adolescence. *Pediatr Hematol Oncol,* **19,** 309-17.
18. Pappo, A.S. (2003) Melanoma in children and adolescents. *Eur J Cancer,* **39,** 2651-61.
19. Marks, R. (2000) Epidemiology of melanoma. *Clin Exp Dermatol,* **25,** 459-63.
20. de Vries, E. and Coebergh, J.W. (2004) Cutaneous malignant melanoma in Europe. *Eur J Cancer,* **40,** 2355-66.
21. Gandini, S., Sera, F., Cattaruzza, M.S., Pasquini, P., Picconi, O., Boyle, P. and Melchi, C.F. (2005) Meta-analysis of risk factors for cutaneous melanoma: II. Sun exposure. *Eur J Cancer,* **41,** 45-60.
22. Elwood, J.M. (1996) Melanoma and sun exposure. *Semin Oncol,* **23,** 650-66.

23. Elwood, J.M. and Jopson, J. (1997) Melanoma and sun exposure: an overview of published studies. *Int J Cancer,* **73,** 198-203.
24. Bliss, J.M., Ford, D., Swerdlow, A.J., Armstrong, B.K., Cristofolini, M., Elwood, J.M., Green, A., Holly, E.A., Mack, T., MacKie, R.M. *et al.* (1995) Risk of cutaneous melanoma associated with pigmentation characteristics and freckling: systematic overview of 10 case-control studies. The International Melanoma Analysis Group (IMAGE). *Int J Cancer,* **62,** 367-76.
25. Noonan, F.P., Recio, J.A., Takayama, H., Duray, P., Anver, M.R., Rush, W.L., De Fabo, E.C. and Merlino, G. (2001) Neonatal sunburn and melanoma in mice. *Nature,* **413,** 271-2.
26. Autier, P. and Dore, J.F. (1998) Influence of sun exposures during childhood and during adulthood on melanoma risk. EPIMEL and EORTC Melanoma Cooperative Group. European Organisation for Research and Treatment of Cancer. *Int J Cancer,* **77,** 533-7.
27. Tucker, M.A., Halpern, A., Holly, E.A., Hartge, P., Elder, D.E., Sagebiel, R.W., Guerry, D.t. and Clark, W.H., Jr. (1997) Clinically recognized dysplastic nevi. A central risk factor for cutaneous melanoma. *Jama,* **277,** 1439-44.
28. Berwick, M. and Halpern, A. (1997) Melanoma epidemiology. *Curr Opin Oncol,* **9,** 178-82.
29. Bauer, J. and Garbe, C. (2003) Acquired melanocytic nevi as risk factor for melanoma development. A comprehensive review of epidemiological data. *Pigment Cell Res,* **16,** 297-306.
30. Grulich, A.E., Bataille, V., Swerdlow, A.J., Newton-Bishop, J.A., Cuzick, J., Hersey, P. and McCarthy, W.H. (1996) Naevi and pigmentary characteristics as risk factors for melanoma in a high-risk population: a case-control study in New South Wales, Australia. *Int J Cancer,* **67,** 485-91.
31. Hayward, N. (2000) New developments in melanoma genetics. *Curr Oncol Rep,* **2,** 300-6.
32. Hayward, N.K. (2003) Genetics of melanoma predisposition. *Oncogene,* **22,** 3053-62.
33. Zuo, L., Weger, J., Yang, Q., Goldstein, A.M., Tucker, M.A., Walker, G.J., Hayward, N. and Dracopoli, N.C. (1996) Germline mutations in the p16INK4a binding domain of CDK4 in familial melanoma. *Nat Genet,* **12,** 97-9.
34. Molven, A., Grimstvedt, M.B., Steine, S.J., Harland, M., Avril, M.F., Hayward, N.K. and Akslen, L.A. (2005) A large Norwegian family with inherited malignant melanoma, multiple atypical nevi, and CDK4 mutation. *Genes Chromosomes Cancer,* **44,** 10-8.
35. Soufir, N., Avril, M.F., Chompret, A., Demenais, F., Bombled, J., Spatz, A., Stoppa-Lyonnet, D., Benard, J. and Bressac-de Paillerets, B. (1998) Prevalence of p16 and CDK4 germline mutations in 48 melanoma-prone families in France. The French Familial Melanoma Study Group. *Hum Mol Genet,* **7,** 209-16.
36. Bevona, C., Goggins, W., Quinn, T., Fullerton, J. and Tsao, H. (2003) Cutaneous melanomas associated with nevi. *Arch Dermatol,* **139,** 1620-4; discussion 1624.
37. Tsao, H., Bevona, C., Goggins, W. and Quinn, T. (2003) The transformation rate of moles (melanocytic nevi) into cutaneous melanoma: a population-based estimate. *Arch Dermatol,* **139,** 282-8.
38. Dore, J.F., Pedeux, R., Boniol, M., Chignol, M.C. and Autier, P. (2001) Intermediate-effect biomarkers in prevention of skin cancer. *IARC Sci Publ,* **154,** 81-91.
39. Hussein, M.R. and Wood, G.S. (2002) Molecular aspects of melanocytic dysplastic nevi. *J Mol Diagn,* **4,** 71-80.
40. Mooi, W.J. (1997) The dysplastic naevus. *J Clin Pathol,* **50,** 711-5.
41. Bennett, D.C. (2003) Human melanocyte senescence and melanoma susceptibility genes. *Oncogene,* **22,** 3063-9.
42. Michaloglou, C., Vredeveld, L.C., Soengas, M.S., Denoyelle, C., Kuilman, T., van der Horst, C.M., Majoor, D.M., Shay, J.W., Mooi, W.J. and Peeper, D.S. (2005) BRAFE600-associated senescence-like cell cycle arrest of human naevi. *Nature,* **436,** 720-4.
43. Clark, W.H. (1991) Tumour progression and the nature of cancer. *Br J Cancer,* **64,** 631-44.

44. Chin, L., Merlino, G. and DePinho, R.A. (1998) Malignant melanoma: modern black plague and genetic black box. *Genes Dev,* **12,** 3467-81.
45. Ivanov, V.N., Bhoumik, A. and Ronai, Z. (2003) Death receptors and melanoma resistance to apoptosis. *Oncogene,* **22,** 3152-61.
46. Balch, C.M., Buzaid, A.C., Soong, S.J., Atkins, M.B., Cascinelli, N., Coit, D.G., Fleming, I.D., Gershenwald, J.E., Houghton, A., Jr., Kirkwood, J.M. et al. (2003) New TNM melanoma staging system: linking biology and natural history to clinical outcomes. *Semin Surg Oncol,* **21,** 43-52.
47. Petro, A., Schwartz, J. and Johnson, T. (2004) Current melanoma staging. *Clin Dermatol,* **22,** 223-7.
48. Lomuto, M., Calabrese, P. and Giuliani, A. (2004) Prognostic signs in melanoma: state of the art. *J Eur Acad Dermatol Venereol,* **18,** 291-300.
49. Lindholm, C., Andersson, R., Dufmats, M., Hansson, J., Ingvar, C., Moller, T., Sjodin, H., Stierner, U. and Wagenius, G. (2004) Invasive cutaneous malignant melanoma in Sweden, 1990-1999. A prospective, population-based study of survival and prognostic factors. *Cancer,* **101,** 2067-78.
50. Meier, S., Baumert, B.G., Maier, T., Wellis, G., Burg, G., Seifert, B. and Dummer, R. (2004) Survival and prognostic factors in patients with brain metastases from malignant melanoma. *Onkologie,* **27,** 145-9.
51. Cuellar, F.A., Vilalta, A., Rull, R., Vidal-Sicart, S., Palou, J., Ventura, P.J., Pous, E., Quinto, L., Malvehy, J., Marti, R. et al. (2004) Small cell melanoma and ulceration as predictors of positive sentinel lymph node in malignant melanoma patients. *Melanoma Res,* **14,** 277-82.
52. Balch, C.M., Soong, S.J., Gershenwald, J.E., Thompson, J.F., Reintgen, D.S., Cascinelli, N., Urist, M., McMasters, K.M., Ross, M.I., Kirkwood, J.M. et al. (2001) Prognostic factors analysis of 17,600 melanoma patients: validation of the American Joint Committee on Cancer melanoma staging system. *J Clin Oncol,* **19,** 3622-34.
53. Balch, C.M., Buzaid, A.C., Soong, S.J., Atkins, M.B., Cascinelli, N., Coit, D.G., Fleming, I.D., Gershenwald, J.E., Houghton, A., Jr., Kirkwood, J.M. et al. (2001) Final version of the American Joint Committee on Cancer staging system for cutaneous melanoma. *J Clin Oncol,* **19,** 3635-48.
54. Sondak, V.K., Taylor, J.M., Sabel, M.S., Wang, Y., Lowe, L., Grover, A.C., Chang, A.E., Yahanda, A.M., Moon, J. and Johnson, T.M. (2004) Mitotic rate and younger age are predictors of sentinel lymph node positivity: lessons learned from the generation of a probabilistic model. *Ann Surg Oncol,* **11,** 247-58.
55. Nagore, E., Oliver, V., Botella-Estrada, R., Moreno-Picot, S., Insa, A. and Fortea, J.M. (2005) Prognostic factors in localized invasive cutaneous melanoma: high value of mitotic rate, vascular invasion and microscopic satellitosis. *Melanoma Res,* **15,** 169-77.
56. Buettner, P.G., Leiter, U., Eigentler, T.K. and Garbe, C. (2005) Development of prognostic factors and survival in cutaneous melanoma over 25 years: An analysis of the Central Malignant Melanoma Registry of the German Dermatological Society. *Cancer,* **103,** 616-24.
57. Hsueh, E.C., Lucci, A., Qi, K. and Morton, D.L. (1999) Survival of patients with melanoma of the lower extremity decreases with distance from the trunk. *Cancer,* **85,** 383-8.
58. Daryanani, D., Plukker, J.T., de Jong, M.A., Haaxma-Reiche, H., Nap, R., Kuiper, H. and Hoekstra, H.J. (2005) Increased incidence of brain metastases in cutaneous head and neck melanoma. *Melanoma Res,* **15,** 119-24.
59. Rockmann, H. and Schadendorf, D. (2003) Drug resistance in human melanoma: mechanisms and therapeutic opportunities. *Onkologie,* **26,** 581-7.
60. Barth, A., Wanek, L.A. and Morton, D.L. (1995) Prognostic factors in 1,521 melanoma patients with distant metastases. *J Am Coll Surg,* **181,** 193-201.
61. Serrano, M., Hannon, G.J. and Beach, D. (1993) A new regulatory motif in cell-cycle control causing specific inhibition of cyclin D/CDK4. *Nature,* **366,** 704-7.

62. Kamb, A., Gruis, N.A., Weaver-Feldhaus, J., Liu, Q., Harshman, K., Tavtigian, S.V., Stockert, E., Day, R.S., 3rd, Johnson, B.E. and Skolnick, M.H. (1994) A cell cycle regulator potentially involved in genesis of many tumor types. *Science,* **264,** 436-40.
63. Nobori, T., Miura, K., Wu, D.J., Lois, A., Takabayashi, K. and Carson, D.A. (1994) Deletions of the cyclin-dependent kinase-4 inhibitor gene in multiple human cancers. *Nature,* **368,** 753-6.
64. Mao, L., Merlo, A., Bedi, G., Shapiro, G.I., Edwards, C.D., Rollins, B.J. and Sidransky, D. (1995) A novel p16INK4A transcript. *Cancer Res,* **55,** 2995-7.
65. Quelle, D.E., Zindy, F., Ashmun, R.A. and Sherr, C.J. (1995) Alternative reading frames of the INK4a tumor suppressor gene encode two unrelated proteins capable of inducing cell cycle arrest. *Cell,* **83,** 993-1000.
66. Liu, L., Goldstein, A.M., Tucker, M.A., Brill, H., Gruis, N.A., Hogg, D. and Lassam, N.J. (1997) Affected members of melanoma-prone families with linkage to 9p21 but lacking mutations in CDKN2A do not harbor mutations in the coding regions of either CDKN2B or p19ARF. *Genes Chromosomes Cancer,* **19,** 52-4.
67. Simon, M., Koster, G., Menon, A.G. and Schramm, J. (1999) Functional evidence for a role of combined CDKN2A (p16-p14(ARF))/CDKN2B (p15) gene inactivation in malignant gliomas. *Acta Neuropathol (Berl),* **98,** 444-52.
68. Ross, J.F., Liu, X. and Dynlacht, B.D. (1999) Mechanism of transcriptional repression of E2F by the retinoblastoma tumor suppressor protein. *Mol Cell,* **3,** 195-205.
69. Harbour, J.W. and Dean, D.C. (2000) The Rb/E2F pathway: expanding roles and emerging paradigms. *Genes Dev,* **14,** 2393-409.
70. Sherr, C.J. (1996) Cancer cell cycles. *Science,* **274,** 1672-7.
71. Tang, K.S., Fersht, A.R. and Itzhaki, L.S. (2003) Sequential unfolding of ankyrin repeats in tumor suppressor p16. *Structure (Camb),* **11,** 67-73.
72. Pomerantz, J., Schreiber-Agus, N., Liegeois, N.J., Silverman, A., Alland, L., Chin, L., Potes, J., Chen, K., Orlow, I., Lee, H.W. *et al.* (1998) The Ink4a tumor suppressor gene product, p19Arf, interacts with MDM2 and neutralizes MDM2's inhibition of p53. *Cell,* **92,** 713-23.
73. Zhang, Y., Xiong, Y. and Yarbrough, W.G. (1998) ARF promotes MDM2 degradation and stabilizes p53: ARF-INK4a locus deletion impairs both the Rb and p53 tumor suppression pathways. *Cell,* **92,** 725-34.
74. Sherr, C.J. and Weber, J.D. (2000) The ARF/p53 pathway. *Curr Opin Genet Dev,* **10,** 94-9.
75. Weber, J.D., Kuo, M.L., Bothner, B., DiGiammarino, E.L., Kriwacki, R.W., Roussel, M.F. and Sherr, C.J. (2000) Cooperative signals governing ARF-mdm2 interaction and nucleolar localization of the complex. *Mol Cell Biol,* **20,** 2517-28.
76. Zhang, Y. and Xiong, Y. (1999) Mutations in human ARF exon 2 disrupt its nucleolar localization and impair its ability to block nuclear export of MDM2 and p53. *Mol Cell,* **3,** 579-91.
77. Tao, W. and Levine, A.J. (1999) P19(ARF) stabilizes p53 by blocking nucleo-cytoplasmic shuttling of Mdm2. *Proc Natl Acad Sci U S A,* **96,** 6937-41.
78. Korgaonkar, C., Zhao, L., Modestou, M. and Quelle, D.E. (2002) ARF function does not require p53 stabilization or Mdm2 relocalization. *Mol Cell Biol,* **22,** 196-206.
79. Llanos, S., Clark, P.A., Rowe, J. and Peters, G. (2001) Stabilization of p53 by p14ARF without relocation of MDM2 to the nucleolus. *Nat Cell Biol,* **3,** 445-52.
80. Zindy, F., Eischen, C.M., Randle, D.H., Kamijo, T., Cleveland, J.L., Sherr, C.J. and Roussel, M.F. (1998) Myc signaling via the ARF tumor suppressor regulates p53-dependent apoptosis and immortalization. *Genes Dev,* **12,** 2424-33.
81. Dimri, G.P., Itahana, K., Acosta, M. and Campisi, J. (2000) Regulation of a senescence checkpoint response by the E2F1 transcription factor and p14(ARF) tumor suppressor. *Mol Cell Biol,* **20,** 273-85.
82. Bates, S., Phillips, A.C., Clark, P.A., Stott, F., Peters, G., Ludwig, R.L. and Vousden, K.H. (1998) p14ARF links the tumour suppressors RB and p53. *Nature,* **395,** 124-5.

83. Palmero, I., Pantoja, C. and Serrano, M. (1998) p19ARF links the tumour suppressor p53 to Ras. *Nature,* **395,** 125-6.
84. Sharpless, N.E., Bardeesy, N., Lee, K.H., Carrasco, D., Castrillon, D.H., Aguirre, A.J., Wu, E.A., Horner, J.W. and DePinho, R.A. (2001) Loss of p16Ink4a with retention of p19Arf predisposes mice to tumorigenesis. *Nature,* **413,** 86-91.
85. Huot, T.J., Rowe, J., Harland, M., Drayton, S., Brookes, S., Gooptu, C., Purkis, P., Fried, M., Bataille, V., Hara, E. *et al.* (2002) Biallelic mutations in p16(INK4a) confer resistance to Ras- and Ets-induced senescence in human diploid fibroblasts. *Mol Cell Biol,* **22,** 8135-43.
86. Kamijo, T., Zindy, F., Roussel, M.F., Quelle, D.E., Downing, J.R., Ashmun, R.A., Grosveld, G. and Sherr, C.J. (1997) Tumor suppression at the mouse INK4a locus mediated by the alternative reading frame product p19ARF. *Cell,* **91,** 649-59.
87. Zindy, F., Quelle, D.E., Roussel, M.F. and Sherr, C.J. (1997) Expression of the p16INK4a tumor suppressor versus other INK4 family members during mouse development and aging. *Oncogene,* **15,** 203-11.
88. Wei, W., Hemmer, R.M. and Sedivy, J.M. (2001) Role of p14(ARF) in replicative and induced senescence of human fibroblasts. *Mol Cell Biol,* **21,** 6748-57.
89. Munro, J., Stott, F.J., Vousden, K.H., Peters, G. and Parkinson, E.K. (1999) Role of the alternative INK4A proteins in human keratinocyte senescence: evidence for the specific inactivation of p16INK4A upon immortalization. *Cancer Res,* **59,** 2516-21.
90. Calabro, V., Mansueto, G., Santoro, R., Gentilella, A., Pollice, A., Ghioni, P., Guerrini, L. and La Mantia, G. (2004) Inhibition of p63 transcriptional activity by p14ARF: functional and physical link between human ARF tumor suppressor and a member of the p53 family. *Mol Cell Biol,* **24,** 8529-40.
91. Suzuki, H., Kurita, M., Mizumoto, K., Moriyama, M., Aiso, S., Nishimoto, I. and Matsuoka, M. (2005) The ARF tumor suppressor inhibits BCL6-mediated transcriptional repression. *Biochem Biophys Res Commun,* **326,** 242-8.
92. Datta, A., Sen, J., Hagen, J., Korgaonkar, C.K., Caffrey, M., Quelle, D.E., Hughes, D.E., Ackerson, T.J., Costa, R.H. and Raychaudhuri, P. (2005) ARF Directly Binds DP1: Interaction with DP1 Coincides with the G1 Arrest Function of ARF. *Mol Cell Biol,* **25,** 8024-36.
93. Ameyar-Zazoua, M., Wisniewska, M.B., Bakiri, L., Wagner, E.F., Yaniv, M. and Weitzman, J.B. (2005) AP-1 dimers regulate transcription of the p14/p19ARF tumor suppressor gene. *Oncogene,* **24,** 2298-306.
94. Rizos, H., Woodruff, S. and Kefford, R.F. (2005) p14ARF interacts with the SUMO-conjugating enzyme Ubc9 and promotes the Sumoylation of its binding partners. *Cell Cycle,* **4,** 597-603.
95. Itahana, K., Bhat, K.P., Jin, A., Itahana, Y., Hawke, D., Kobayashi, R. and Zhang, Y. (2003) Tumor suppressor ARF degrades B23, a nucleolar protein involved in ribosome biogenesis and cell proliferation. *Mol Cell,* **12,** 1151-64.
96. Sugimoto, M., Kuo, M.L., Roussel, M.F. and Sherr, C.J. (2003) Nucleolar Arf tumor suppressor inhibits ribosomal RNA processing. *Mol Cell,* **11,** 415-24.
97. Maeda, T., Hobbs, R.M., Merghoub, T., Guernah, I., Zelent, A., Cordon-Cardo, C., Teruya-Feldstein, J. and Pandolfi, P.P. (2005) Role of the proto-oncogene Pokemon in cellular transformation and ARF repression. *Nature,* **433,** 278-85.
98. Jacobs, J.J., Keblusek, P., Robanus-Maandag, E., Kristel, P., Lingbeek, M., Nederlof, P.M., van Welsem, T., van de Vijver, M.J., Koh, E.Y., Daley, G.Q. *et al.* (2000) Senescence bypass screen identifies TBX2, which represses Cdkn2a (p19(ARF)) and is amplified in a subset of human breast cancers. *Nat Genet,* **26,** 291-9.
99. Maestro, R., Dei Tos, A.P., Hamamori, Y., Krasnokutsky, S., Sartorelli, V., Kedes, L., Doglioni, C., Beach, D.H. and Hannon, G.J. (1999) Twist is a potential oncogene that inhibits apoptosis. *Genes Dev,* **13,** 2207-17.

100. Serrano, M., Lee, H., Chin, L., Cordon-Cardo, C., Beach, D. and DePinho, R.A. (1996) Role of the INK4a locus in tumor suppression and cell mortality. *Cell*, **85**, 27-37.
101. Krimpenfort, P., Quon, K.C., Mooi, W.J., Loonstra, A. and Berns, A. (2001) Loss of p16Ink4a confers susceptibility to metastatic melanoma in mice. *Nature*, **413**, 83-6.
102. Chin, L., Pomerantz, J., Polsky, D., Jacobson, M., Cohen, C., Cordon-Cardo, C., Horner, J.W., 2nd and DePinho, R.A. (1997) Cooperative effects of INK4a and ras in melanoma susceptibility in vivo. *Genes Dev*, **11**, 2822-34.
103. Koenig, A., Bianco, S.R., Fosmire, S., Wojcieszyn, J. and Modiano, J.F. (2002) Expression and significance of p53, rb, p21/waf-1, p16/ink-4a, and PTEN tumor suppressors in canine melanoma. *Vet Pathol*, **39**, 458-72.
104. Levine, R.A. and Fleischli, M.A. (2000) Inactivation of p53 and retinoblastoma family pathways in canine osteosarcoma cell lines. *Vet Pathol*, **37**, 54-61.
105. Belinsky, S.A., Nikula, K.J., Palmisano, W.A., Michels, R., Saccomanno, G., Gabrielson, E., Baylin, S.B. and Herman, J.G. (1998) Aberrant methylation of p16(INK4a) is an early event in lung cancer and a potential biomarker for early diagnosis. *Proc Natl Acad Sci U S A*, **95**, 11891-6.
106. Schlegel, J., Piontek, G., Kersting, M., Schuermann, M., Kappler, R., Scherthan, H., Weghorst, C., Buzard, G. and Mennel, H. (1999) The p16/Cdkn2a/Ink4a gene is frequently deleted in nitrosourea-induced rat glial tumors. *Pathobiology*, **67**, 202-6.
107. Nairn, R.S., Kazianis, S., McEntire, B.B., Della Coletta, L., Walter, R.B. and Morizot, D.C. (1996) A CDKN2-like polymorphism in Xiphophorus LG V is associated with UV-B-induced melanoma formation in platyfish-swordtail hybrids. *Proc Natl Acad Sci U S A*, **93**, 13042-7.
108. Hemminki, K., Lonnstedt, I., Vaittinen, P. and Lichtenstein, P. (2001) Estimation of genetic and environmental components in colorectal and lung cancer and melanoma. *Genet Epidemiol*, **20**, 107-116.
109. Lichtenstein, P., Holm, N.V., Verkasalo, P.K., Iliadou, A., Kaprio, J., Koskenvuo, M., Pukkala, E., Skytthe, A. and Hemminki, K. (2000) Environmental and heritable factors in the causation of cancer--analyses of cohorts of twins from Sweden, Denmark, and Finland. *N Engl J Med*, **343**, 78-85.
110. Hemminki, K., Lonnstedt, I. and Vaittinen, P. (2001) A population-based study of familial cutaneous melanoma. *Melanoma Res*, **11**, 133-40.
111. Bishop, D.T., Demenais, F., Goldstein, A.M., Bergman, W., Bishop, J.N., Bressac-de Paillerets, B., Chompret, A., Ghiorzo, P., Gruis, N., Hansson, J. *et al.* (2002) Geographical variation in the penetrance of CDKN2A mutations for melanoma. *J Natl Cancer Inst*, **94**, 894-903.
112. Bressac-de-Paillerets, B., Avril, M.F., Chompret, A. and Demenais, F. (2002) Genetic and environmental factors in cutaneous malignant melanoma. *Biochimie*, **84**, 67-74.
113. Goldstein, A.M., Struewing, J.P., Chidambaram, A., Fraser, M.C. and Tucker, M.A. (2000) Genotype-phenotype relationships in U.S. melanoma-prone families with CDKN2A and CDK4 mutations. *J Natl Cancer Inst*, **92**, 1006-10.
114. Lal, G., Liu, L., Hogg, D., Lassam, N.J., Redston, M.S. and Gallinger, S. (2000) Patients with both pancreatic adenocarcinoma and melanoma may harbor germline CDKN2A mutations. *Genes Chromosomes Cancer*, **27**, 358-61.
115. Kumar, R., Sauroja, I., Punnonen, K., Jansen, C. and Hemminki, K. (1998) Selective deletion of exon 1 beta of the p19ARF gene in metastatic melanoma cell lines. *Genes Chromosomes Cancer*, **23**, 273-7.
116. Mistry, S.H., Taylor, C., Randerson-Moor, J.A., Harland, M., Turner, F., Barrett, J.H., Whitaker, L., Jenkins, R.B., Knowles, M.A., Bishop, J.A. *et al.* (2005) Prevalence of 9p21 deletions in UK melanoma families. *Genes Chromosomes Cancer*.
117. Bahuau, M., Vidaud, D., Kujas, M., Palangie, A., Assouline, B., Chaignaud-Lebreton, M., Prieur, M., Vidaud, M., Harpey, J.P., Lafourcade, J. *et al.* (1997) Familial aggregation of

malignant melanoma/dysplastic naevi and tumours of the nervous system: an original syndrome of tumour proneness. *Ann Genet,* **40,** 78-91.
118. Petronzelli, F., Sollima, D., Coppola, G., Martini-Neri, M.E., Neri, G. and Genuardi, M. (2001) CDKN2A germline splicing mutation affecting both p16(ink4) and p14(arf) RNA processing in a melanoma/neurofibroma kindred. *Genes Chromosomes Cancer,* **31,** 398-401.
119. Randerson-Moor, J.A., Harland, M., Williams, S., Cuthbert-Heavens, D., Sheridan, E., Aveyard, J., Sibley, K., Whitaker, L., Knowles, M., Bishop, J.N. *et al.* (2001) A germline deletion of p14(ARF) but not CDKN2A in a melanoma-neural system tumour syndrome family. *Hum Mol Genet,* **10,** 55-62.
120. Quelle, D.E., Cheng, M., Ashmun, R.A. and Sherr, C.J. (1997) Cancer-associated mutations at the INK4a locus cancel cell cycle arrest by p16INK4a but not by the alternative reading frame protein p19ARF. *Proc Natl Acad Sci U S A,* **94,** 669-73.
121. Hewitt, C., Lee Wu, C., Evans, G., Howell, A., Elles, R.G., Jordan, R., Sloan, P., Read, A.P. and Thakker, N. (2002) Germline mutation of ARF in a melanoma kindred. *Hum Mol Genet,* **11,** 1273-9.
122. Rizos, H., Puig, S., Badenas, C., Malvehy, J., Darmanian, A.P., Jimenez, L., Mila, M. and Kefford, R.F. (2001) A melanoma-associated germline mutation in exon 1beta inactivates p14ARF. *Oncogene,* **20,** 5543-7.
123. Harland, M., Taylor, C.F., Chambers, P.A., Kukalizch, K., Randerson-Moor, J.A., Gruis, N.A., de Snoo, F.A., ter Huurne, J.A., Goldstein, A.M., Tucker, M.A. *et al.* (2005) A mutation hotspot at the p14ARF splice site. *Oncogene,* **24,** 4604-8.
124. Flores, J.F., Walker, G.J., Glendening, J.M., Haluska, F.G., Castresana, J.S., Rubio, M.P., Pastorfide, G.C., Boyer, L.A., Kao, W.H., Bulyk, M.L. *et al.* (1996) Loss of the p16INK4a and p15INK4b genes, as well as neighboring 9p21 markers, in sporadic melanoma. *Cancer Res,* **56,** 5023-32.
125. Walker, G.J., Flores, J.F., Glendening, J.M., Lin, A.H., Markl, I.D. and Fountain, J.W. (1998) Virtually 100% of melanoma cell lines harbor alterations at the DNA level within CDKN2A, CDKN2B, or one of their downstream targets. *Genes Chromosomes Cancer,* **22,** 157-63.
126. Kumar, R., Lundh Rozell, B., Louhelainen, J. and Hemminki, K. (1998) Mutations in the CDKN2A (p16INK4a) gene in microdissected sporadic primary melanomas. *Int J Cancer,* **75,** 193-8.
127. Fujimoto, A., Morita, R., Hatta, N., Takehara, K. and Takata, M. (1999) p16INK4a inactivation is not frequent in uncultured sporadic primary cutaneous melanoma. *Oncogene,* **18,** 2527-32.
128. Alao, J.P., Mohammed, M.Q. and Retsas, S. (2002) The CDKN2A tumour suppressor gene: no mutations detected in patients with melanoma and additional unrelated cancers. *Melanoma Res,* **12,** 559-63.
129. Rocco, J.W. and Sidransky, D. (2001) p16(MTS-1/CDKN2/INK4a) in cancer progression. *Exp Cell Res,* **264,** 42-55.
130. Gonzalgo, M.L., Bender, C.M., You, E.H., Glendening, J.M., Flores, J.F., Walker, G.J., Hayward, N.K., Jones, P.A. and Fountain, J.W. (1997) Low frequency of p16/CDKN2A methylation in sporadic melanoma: comparative approaches for methylation analysis of primary tumors. *Cancer Res,* **57,** 5336-47.
131. von Eggeling, F., Werner, G., Theuer, C., Riese, U., Dahse, R., Fiedler, W., Schimmel, B., Ernst, G., Karte, K., Claussen, U. *et al.* (1999) Analysis of the tumor suppressor gene p16(INK4A) in microdissected melanoma metastases by sequencing, and microsatellite and methylation screening. *Arch Dermatol Res,* **291,** 474-7.
132. Cachia, A.R., Indsto, J.O., McLaren, K.M., Mann, G.J. and Arends, M.J. (2000) CDKN2A mutation and deletion status in thin and thick primary melanoma. *Clin Cancer Res,* **6,** 3511-5.

133. Kumar, R., Smeds, J., Lundh Rozell, B. and Hemminki, K. (1999) Loss of heterozygosity at chromosome 9p21 (INK4-p14ARF locus): homozygous deletions and mutations in the p16 and p14ARF genes in sporadic primary melanomas. *Melanoma Res*, **9**, 138-47.
134. Smeds, J., Kumar, R., Rozell, B.L. and Hemminki, K. (2000) Increased frequency of LOH on chromosome 9 in sporadic primary melanomas is associated with increased patient age at diagnosis. *Mutagenesis*, **15**, 257-60.
135. Pollock, P.M., Welch, J. and Hayward, N.K. (2001) Evidence for three tumor suppressor loci on chromosome 9p involved in melanoma development. *Cancer Res*, **61**, 1154-61.
136. Pavey, S.J., Cummings, M.C., Whiteman, D.C., Castellano, M., Walsh, M.D., Gabrielli, B.G., Green, A. and Hayward, N.K. (2002) Loss of p16 expression is associated with histological features of melanoma invasion. *Melanoma Res*, **12**, 539-47.
137. Straume, O., Sviland, L. and Akslen, L.A. (2000) Loss of nuclear p16 protein expression correlates with increased tumor cell proliferation (Ki-67) and poor prognosis in patients with vertical growth phase melanoma. *Clin Cancer Res*, **6**, 1845-53.
138. Lamperska, K., Mackiewicz, K., Kaczmarek, A., Kwiatkowska, E., Starzycka, M., Romanowska, B., Heizman, J., Stachura, J. and Mackiewicz, A. (2002) Expression of p16 in sporadic primary uveal melanoma. *Acta Biochim Pol*, **49**, 377-85.
139. Aitken, J., Welch, J., Duffy, D., Milligan, A., Green, A., Martin, N. and Hayward, N. (1999) CDKN2A variants in a population-based sample of Queensland families with melanoma. *J Natl Cancer Inst*, **91**, 446-52.
140. Kumar, R., Smeds, J., Berggren, P., Straume, O., Rozell, B.L., Akslen, L.A. and Hemminki, K. (2001) A single nucleotide polymorphism in the 3'untranslated region of the CDKN2A gene is common in sporadic primary melanomas but mutations in the CDKN2B, CDKN2C, CDK4 and p53 genes are rare. *Int J Cancer*, **95**, 388-93.
141. Chaubert, P., Shaw, P. and Pillet, N. (1996) Informative MspI polymorphism adjacent to exon 3 of the p16INK4 (MTS1) gene. *Mol Cell Probes*, **10**, 467-8.
142. Holland, E.A., Beaton, S.C., Becker, T.M., Grulet, O.M., Peters, B.A., Rizos, H., Kefford, R.F. and Mann, G.J. (1995) Analysis of the p16 gene, CDKN2, in 17 Australian melanoma kindreds. *Oncogene*, **11**, 2289-94.
143. Sauroja, I., Smeds, J., Vlaykova, T., Kumar, R., Talve, L., Hahka-Kemppinen, M., Punnonen, K., Jansen, C.T., Hemminki, K. and Pyrhonen, S. (2000) Analysis of G(1)/S checkpoint regulators in metastatic melanoma. *Genes Chromosomes Cancer*, **28**, 404-14.
144. Straume, O., Smeds, J., Kumar, R., Hemminki, K. and Akslen, L.A. (2002) Significant impact of promoter hypermethylation and the 540 C>T polymorphism of CDKN2A in cutaneous melanoma of the vertical growth phase. *Am J Pathol*, **161**, 229-37.
145. Lilischkis, R., Sarcevic, B., Kennedy, C., Warlters, A. and Sutherland, R.L. (1996) Cancer-associated mis-sense and deletion mutations impair p16INK4 CDK inhibitory activity. *Int J Cancer*, **66**, 249-54.
146. Ruas, M. and Peters, G. (1998) The p16INK4a/CDKN2A tumor suppressor and its relatives. *Biochim Biophys Acta*, **1378**, F115-77.
147. Reymond, A. and Brent, R. (1995) p16 proteins from melanoma-prone families are deficient in binding to Cdk4. *Oncogene*, **11**, 1173-8.
148. Debniak, T., Scott, R.J., Huzarski, T., Byrski, T., Rozmiarek, A., Debniak, B., Zaluga, E., Maleszka, R., Kladny, J., Gorski, B. *et al.* (2005) CDKN2A common variants and their association with melanoma risk: a population-based study. *Cancer Res*, **65**, 835-9.
149. Puig, S., Malvehy, J., Badenas, C., Ruiz, A., Jimenez, D., Cuellar, F., Azon, A., Gonzalez, U., Castel, T., Campoy, A. *et al.* (2005) Role of the CDKN2A locus in patients with multiple primary melanomas. *J Clin Oncol*, **23**, 3043-51.
150. Sharpless, E. and Chin, L. (2003) The INK4a/ARF locus and melanoma. *Oncogene*, **22**, 3092-8.
151. Greenblatt, M.S., Beaudet, J.G., Gump, J.R., Godin, K.S., Trombley, L., Koh, J. and Bond, J.P. (2003) Detailed computational study of p53 and p16: using evolutionary sequence

analysis and disease-associated mutations to predict the functional consequences of allelic variants. *Oncogene,* **22,** 1150-63.
152. Yang, R., Gombart, A.F., Serrano, M. and Koeffler, H.P. (1995) Mutational effects on the p16INK4a tumor suppressor protein. *Cancer Res,* **55,** 2503-6.
153. Caldas, C., Hahn, S.A., da Costa, L.T., Redston, M.S., Schutte, M., Seymour, A.B., Weinstein, C.L., Hruban, R.H., Yeo, C.J. and Kern, S.E. (1994) Frequent somatic mutations and homozygous deletions of the p16 (MTS1) gene in pancreatic adenocarcinoma. *Nat Genet,* **8,** 27-32.
154. Maesawa, C., Tamura, G., Nishizuka, S., Ogasawara, S., Ishida, K., Terashima, M., Sakata, K., Sato, N., Saito, K. and Satodate, R. (1996) Inactivation of the CDKN2 gene by homozygous deletion and de novo methylation is associated with advanced stage esophageal squamous cell carcinoma. *Cancer Res,* **56,** 3875-8.
155. Ragione, F.D. and Iolascon, A. (1997) Inactivation of cyclin-dependent kinase inhibitor genes and development of human acute leukemias. *Leuk Lymphoma,* **25,** 23-35.
156. Reed, A.L., Califano, J., Cairns, P., Westra, W.H., Jones, R.M., Koch, W., Ahrendt, S., Eby, Y., Sewell, D., Nawroz, H. *et al.* (1996) High frequency of p16 (CDKN2/MTS-1/INK4A) inactivation in head and neck squamous cell carcinoma. *Cancer Res,* **56,** 3630-3.
157. Marsit, C.J., Karagas, M.R., Danaee, H., Liu, M., Andrew, A., Schned, A., Nelson, H.H. and Kelsey, K.T. (2005) Carcinogen exposure and gene promoter hypermethylation in bladder cancer. *Carcinogenesis.*
158. Breuer, R.H., Snijders, P.J., Sutedja, G.T., Sewalt, R.G., Otte, A.P., Postmus, P.E., Meijer, C.J., Raaphorst, F.M. and Smit, E.F. (2005) Expression of the p16(INK4a) gene product, methylation of the p16(INK4a) promoter region and expression of the polycomb-group gene BMI-1 in squamous cell lung carcinoma and premalignant endobronchial lesions. *Lung Cancer,* **48,** 299-306.
159. Hou, P., Ji, M.J., Shen, J.Y., He, N.Y. and Lu, Z.H. (2005) Detection of p16 hypermethylation in gastric carcinomas using a seminested methylation-specific PCR. *Biochem Genet,* **43,** 1-9.
160. Schildhaus, H.U., Krockel, I., Lippert, H., Malfertheiner, P., Roessner, A. and Schneider-Stock, R. (2005) Promoter hypermethylation of p16INK4a, E-cadherin, O6-MGMT, DAPK and FHIT in adenocarcinomas of the esophagus, esophagogastric junction and proximal stomach. *Int J Oncol,* **26,** 1493-500.
161. Gardie, B., Cayuela, J.M., Martini, S. and Sigaux, F. (1998) Genomic alterations of the p19ARF encoding exons in T-cell acute lymphoblastic leukemia. *Blood,* **91,** 1016-20.
162. Zhang, S.J., Endo, S., Saito, T., Kouno, M., Kuroiwa, T., Washiyama, K. and Kumanishi, T. (2005) Primary malignant lymphoma of the brain: frequent abnormalities and inactivation of p14 tumor suppressor gene. *Cancer Sci,* **96,** 38-41.
163. Smeds, J., Berggren, P., Ma, X., Xu, Z., Hemminki, K. and Kumar, R. (2002) Genetic status of cell cycle regulators in squamous cell carcinoma of the oesophagus: the CDKN2A (p16(INK4a) and p14(ARF)) and p53 genes are major targets for inactivation. *Carcinogenesis,* **23,** 645-55.
164. Sato, F., Harpaz, N., Shibata, D., Xu, Y., Yin, J., Mori, Y., Zou, T.T., Wang, S., Desai, K., Leytin, A. *et al.* (2002) Hypermethylation of the p14(ARF) gene in ulcerative colitis-associated colorectal carcinogenesis. *Cancer Res,* **62,** 1148-51.
165. Anzola, M., Cuevas, N., Lopez-Martinez, M., Saiz, A., Burgos, J.J. and Martinez de Pancorboa, M. (2004) P14ARF gene alterations in human hepatocellular carcinoma. *Eur J Gastroenterol Hepatol,* **16,** 19-26.
166. Iida, S., Akiyama, Y., Nakajima, T., Ichikawa, W., Nihei, Z., Sugihara, K. and Yuasa, Y. (2000) Alterations and hypermethylation of the p14(ARF) gene in gastric cancer. *Int J Cancer,* **87,** 654-8.

167. Nakamura, M., Watanabe, T., Klangby, U., Asker, C., Wiman, K., Yonekawa, Y., Kleihues, P. and Ohgaki, H. (2001) p14ARF deletion and methylation in genetic pathways to glioblastomas. *Brain Pathol*, **11**, 159-68.
168. Maher, E.A., Furnari, F.B., Bachoo, R.M., Rowitch, D.H., Louis, D.N., Cavenee, W.K. and DePinho, R.A. (2001) Malignant glioma: genetics and biology of a grave matter. *Genes Dev*, **15**, 1311-33.
169. Ortega, S., Malumbres, M. and Barbacid, M. (2002) Cyclin D-dependent kinases, INK4 inhibitors and cancer. *Biochim Biophys Acta*, **1602**, 73-87.
170. Rane, S.G., Dubus, P., Mettus, R.V., Galbreath, E.J., Boden, G., Reddy, E.P. and Barbacid, M. (1999) Loss of Cdk4 expression causes insulin-deficient diabetes and Cdk4 activation results in beta-islet cell hyperplasia. *Nat Genet*, **22**, 44-52.
171. Sotillo, R., Garcia, J.F., Ortega, S., Martin, J., Dubus, P., Barbacid, M. and Malumbres, M. (2001) Invasive melanoma in Cdk4-targeted mice. *Proc Natl Acad Sci U S A*, **98**, 13312-7.
172. Cohen, Y., Goldenberg-Cohen, N., Parrella, P., Chowers, I., Merbs, S.L., Pe'er, J. and Sidransky, D. (2003) Lack of BRAF mutation in primary uveal melanoma. *Invest Ophthalmol Vis Sci*, **44**, 2876-8.
173. Satyamoorthy, K., Li, G., Gerrero, M.R., Brose, M.S., Volpe, P., Weber, B.L., Van Belle, P., Elder, D.E. and Herlyn, M. (2003) Constitutive mitogen-activated protein kinase activation in melanoma is mediated by both BRAF mutations and autocrine growth factor stimulation. *Cancer Res*, **63**, 756-9.
174. Smalley, K.S. (2003) A pivotal role for ERK in the oncogenic behaviour of malignant melanoma? *Int J Cancer*, **104**, 527-32.
175. Wellbrock, C., Karasarides, M. and Marais, R. (2004) The RAF proteins take centre stage. *Nat Rev Mol Cell Biol*, **5**, 875-85.
176. Pouyssegur, J. and Lenormand, P. (2003) Fidelity and spatio-temporal control in MAP kinase (ERKs) signalling. *Eur J Biochem*, **270**, 3291-9.
177. Sebolt-Leopold, J.S. and Herrera, R. (2004) Targeting the mitogen-activated protein kinase cascade to treat cancer. *Nat Rev Cancer*, **4**, 937-47.
178. Busca, R., Abbe, P., Mantoux, F., Aberdam, E., Peyssonnaux, C., Eychene, A., Ortonne, J.P. and Ballotti, R. (2000) Ras mediates the cAMP-dependent activation of extracellular signal-regulated kinases (ERKs) in melanocytes. *Embo J*, **19**, 2900-10.
179. Dumaz, N. and Marais, R. (2005) Integrating signals between cAMP and the RAS/RAF/MEK/ERK signalling pathways. *Febs J*, **272**, 3491-504.
180. Pruitt, K. and Der, C.J. (2001) Ras and Rho regulation of the cell cycle and oncogenesis. *Cancer Lett*, **171**, 1-10.
181. Schulze, A., Lehmann, K., Jefferies, H.B., McMahon, M. and Downward, J. (2001) Analysis of the transcriptional program induced by Raf in epithelial cells. *Genes Dev*, **15**, 981-94.
182. Huntington, J.T., Shields, J.M., Der, C.J., Wyatt, C.A., Benbow, U., Slingluff, C.L., Jr. and Brinckerhoff, C.E. (2004) Overexpression of collagenase 1 (MMP-1) is mediated by the ERK pathway in invasive melanoma cells: role of BRAF mutation and fibroblast growth factor signaling. *J Biol Chem*, **279**, 33168-76.
183. Woods, D., Cherwinski, H., Venetsanakos, E., Bhat, A., Gysin, S., Humbert, M., Bray, P.F., Saylor, V.L. and McMahon, M. (2001) Induction of beta3-integrin gene expression by sustained activation of the Ras-regulated Raf-MEK-extracellular signal-regulated kinase signaling pathway. *Mol Cell Biol*, **21**, 3192-205.
184. Campbell, P.M. and Der, C.J. (2004) Oncogenic Ras and its role in tumor cell invasion and metastasis. *Semin Cancer Biol*, **14**, 105-14.
185. Morrison, D.K. and Cutler, R.E. (1997) The complexity of Raf-1 regulation. *Curr Opin Cell Biol*, **9**, 174-9.
186. Mercer, K.E. and Pritchard, C.A. (2003) Raf proteins and cancer: B-Raf is identified as a mutational target. *Biochim Biophys Acta*, **1653**, 25-40.

187. Wojnowski, L., Zimmer, A.M., Beck, T.W., Hahn, H., Bernal, R., Rapp, U.R. and Zimmer, A. (1997) Endothelial apoptosis in Braf-deficient mice. *Nat Genet,* **16,** 293-7.
188. Wojnowski, L., Stancato, L.F., Zimmer, A.M., Hahn, H., Beck, T.W., Larner, A.C., Rapp, U.R. and Zimmer, A. (1998) Craf-1 protein kinase is essential for mouse development. *Mech Dev,* **76,** 141-9.
189. Pritchard, C.A., Bolin, L., Slattery, R., Murray, R. and McMahon, M. (1996) Post-natal lethality and neurological and gastrointestinal defects in mice with targeted disruption of the A-Raf protein kinase gene. *Curr Biol,* **6,** 614-7.
190. Storm, S.M., Cleveland, J.L. and Rapp, U.R. (1990) Expression of raf family proto-oncogenes in normal mouse tissues. *Oncogene,* **5,** 345-51.
191. Chong, H., Vikis, H.G. and Guan, K.L. (2003) Mechanisms of regulating the Raf kinase family. *Cell Signal,* **15,** 463-9.
192. Barnier, J.V., Papin, C., Eychene, A., Lecoq, O. and Calothy, G. (1995) The mouse B-raf gene encodes multiple protein isoforms with tissue-specific expression. *J Biol Chem,* **270,** 23381-9.
193. Davies, H., Bignell, G.R., Cox, C., Stephens, P., Edkins, S., Clegg, S., Teague, J., Woffendin, H., Garnett, M.J., Bottomley, W. *et al.* (2002) Mutations of the BRAF gene in human cancer. *Nature,* **417,** 949-54.
194. Garnett, M.J. and Marais, R. (2004) Guilty as charged: B-RAF is a human oncogene. *Cancer Cell,* **6,** 313-9.
195. Wan, P.T., Garnett, M.J., Roe, S.M., Lee, S., Niculescu-Duvaz, D., Good, V.M., Jones, C.M., Marshall, C.J., Springer, C.J., Barford, D. *et al.* (2004) Mechanism of activation of the RAF-ERK signaling pathway by oncogenic mutations of B-RAF. *Cell,* **116,** 855-67.
196. Gray-Schopfer, V.C., da Rocha Dias, S. and Marais, R. (2005) The role of B-RAF in melanoma. *Cancer Metastasis Rev,* **24,** 165-83.
197. Kumar, R., Angelini, S. and Hemminki, K. (2003) Activating BRAF and N-Ras mutations in sporadic primary melanomas: an inverse association with allelic loss on chromosome 9. *Oncogene,* **22,** 9217-24.
198. Brose, M.S., Volpe, P., Feldman, M., Kumar, M., Rishi, I., Gerrero, R., Einhorn, E., Herlyn, M., Minna, J., Nicholson, A. *et al.* (2002) BRAF and RAS mutations in human lung cancer and melanoma. *Cancer Res,* **62,** 6997-7000.
199. Omholt, K., Platz, A., Kanter, L., Ringborg, U. and Hansson, J. (2003) NRAS and BRAF mutations arise early during melanoma pathogenesis and are preserved throughout tumor progression. *Clin Cancer Res,* **9,** 6483-8.
200. Pollock, P.M., Harper, U.L., Hansen, K.S., Yudt, L.M., Stark, M., Robbins, C.M., Moses, T.Y., Hostetter, G., Wagner, U., Kakareka, J. *et al.* (2003) High frequency of BRAF mutations in nevi. *Nat Genet,* **33,** 19-20.
201. Saldanha, G., Purnell, D., Fletcher, A., Potter, L., Gillies, A. and Pringle, J.H. (2004) High BRAF mutation frequency does not characterize all melanocytic tumor types. *Int J Cancer,* **111,** 705-10.
202. Kumar, R., Angelini, S., Snellman, E. and Hemminki, K. (2004) BRAF mutations are common somatic events in melanocytic nevi. *J Invest Dermatol,* **122,** 342-8.
203. Yazdi, A.S., Palmedo, G., Flaig, M.J., Puchta, U., Reckwerth, A., Rutten, A., Mentzel, T., Hugel, H., Hantschke, M., Schmid-Wendtner, M.H. *et al.* (2003) Mutations of the BRAF gene in benign and malignant melanocytic lesions. *J Invest Dermatol,* **121,** 1160-2.
204. Patton, E.E., Widlund, H.R., Kutok, J.L., Kopani, K.R., Amatruda, J.F., Murphey, R.D., Berghmans, S., Mayhall, E.A., Traver, D., Fletcher, C.D. *et al.* (2005) BRAF mutations are sufficient to promote nevi formation and cooperate with p53 in the genesis of melanoma. *Curr Biol,* **15,** 249-54.
205. Wellbrock, C., Ogilvie, L., Hedley, D., Karasarides, M., Martin, J., Niculescu-Duvaz, D., Springer, C.J. and Marais, R. (2004) V599EB-RAF is an oncogene in melanocytes. *Cancer Res,* **64,** 2338-42.

206. Sumimoto, H., Miyagishi, M., Miyoshi, H., Yamagata, S., Shimizu, A., Taira, K. and Kawakami, Y. (2004) Inhibition of growth and invasive ability of melanoma by inactivation of mutated BRAF with lentivirus-mediated RNA interference. *Oncogene,* **23,** 6031-9.
207. Sharma, A., Trivedi, N.R., Zimmerman, M.A., Tuveson, D.A., Smith, C.D. and Robertson, G.P. (2005) Mutant V599EB-Raf regulates growth and vascular development of malignant melanoma tumors. *Cancer Res,* **65,** 2412-21.
208. Bhatt, K.V., Spofford, L.S., Aram, G., McMullen, M., Pumiglia, K. and Aplin, A.E. (2005) Adhesion control of cyclin D1 and p27Kip1 levels is deregulated in melanoma cells through BRAF-MEK-ERK signaling. *Oncogene,* **24,** 3459-71.
209. Smalley, K.S. and Herlyn, M. (2004) Loitering with intent: new evidence for the role of BRAF mutations in the proliferation of melanocytic lesions. *J Invest Dermatol,* **123,** xvi-xvii.
210. Zuidervaart, W., van Nieuwpoort, F., Stark, M., Dijkman, R., Packer, L., Borgstein, A.M., Pavey, S., van der Velden, P., Out, C., Jager, M.J. *et al.* (2005) Activation of the MAPK pathway is a common event in uveal melanomas although it rarely occurs through mutation of BRAF or RAS. *Br J Cancer,* **92,** 2032-8.
211. Cruz, F., 3rd, Rubin, B.P., Wilson, D., Town, A., Schroeder, A., Haley, A., Bainbridge, T., Heinrich, M.C. and Corless, C.L. (2003) Absence of BRAF and NRAS mutations in uveal melanoma. *Cancer Res,* **63,** 5761-6.
212. Ciampi, R., Knauf, J.A., Kerler, R., Gandhi, M., Zhu, Z., Nikiforova, M.N., Rabes, H.M., Fagin, J.A. and Nikiforov, Y.E. (2005) Oncogenic AKAP9-BRAF fusion is a novel mechanism of MAPK pathway activation in thyroid cancer. *J Clin Invest,* **115,** 94-101.
213. Barbacid, M. (1987) ras genes. *Annu Rev Biochem,* **56,** 779-827.
214. Silvius, J.R. (2002) Mechanisms of Ras protein targeting in mammalian cells. *J Membr Biol,* **190,** 83-92.
215. Bos, J.L. (1989) ras oncogenes in human cancer: a review. *Cancer Res,* **49,** 4682-9.
216. Der, C.J., Finkel, T. and Cooper, G.M. (1986) Biological and biochemical properties of human rasH genes mutated at codon 61. *Cell,* **44,** 167-76.
217. Polakis, P. and McCormick, F. (1993) Structural requirements for the interaction of p21ras with GAP, exchange factors, and its biological effector target. *J Biol Chem,* **268,** 9157-60.
218. Omholt, K., Karsberg, S., Platz, A., Kanter, L., Ringborg, U. and Hansson, J. (2002) Screening of N-ras codon 61 mutations in paired primary and metastatic cutaneous melanomas: mutations occur early and persist throughout tumor progression. *Clin Cancer Res,* **8,** 3468-74.
219. Demunter, A., Stas, M., Degreef, H., De Wolf-Peeters, C. and van den Oord, J.J. (2001) Analysis of N- and K-ras mutations in the distinctive tumor progression phases of melanoma. *J Invest Dermatol,* **117,** 1483-9.
220. Papp, T., Pemsel, H., Zimmermann, R., Bastrop, R., Weiss, D.G. and Schiffmann, D. (1999) Mutational analysis of N-ras, p53, p16INK4a, CDK4, and MC1R genes in human congenital melanocytic naevi. *J Med Genet,* **36,** 610-4.
221. van 't Veer, L.J., Burgering, B.M., Versteeg, R., Boot, A.J., Ruiter, D.J., Osanto, S., Schrier, P.I. and Bos, J.L. (1989) N-ras mutations in human cutaneous melanoma from sun-exposed body sites. *Mol Cell Biol,* **9,** 3114-6.
222. van Elsas, A., Zerp, S.F., van der Flier, S., Kruse, K.M., Aarnoudse, C., Hayward, N.K., Ruiter, D.J. and Schrier, P.I. (1996) Relevance of ultraviolet-induced N-ras oncogene point mutations in development of primary human cutaneous melanoma. *Am J Pathol,* **149,** 883-93.
223. Jiveskog, S., Ragnarsson-Olding, B., Platz, A. and Ringborg, U. (1998) N-ras mutations are common in melanomas from sun-exposed skin of humans but rare in mucosal membranes or unexposed skin. *J Invest Dermatol,* **111,** 757-61.

224. Eskandarpour, M., Kiaii, S., Zhu, C., Castro, J., Sakko, A.J. and Hansson, J. (2005) Suppression of oncogenic NRAS by RNA interference induces apoptosis of human melanoma cells. *Int J Cancer*, **115**, 65-73.
225. Garraway, L.A., Widlund, H.R., Rubin, M.A., Getz, G., Berger, A.J., Ramaswamy, S., Beroukhim, R., Milner, D.A., Granter, S.R., Du, J. *et al.* (2005) Integrative genomic analyses identify MITF as a lineage survival oncogene amplified in malignant melanoma. *Nature*, **436**, 117-22.
226. Ackermann, J., Frutschi, M., Kaloulis, K., McKee, T., Trumpp, A. and Beermann, F. (2005) Metastasizing melanoma formation caused by expression of activated N-RasQ61K on an INK4a-deficient background. *Cancer Res*, **65**, 4005-11.
227. Golub, T.R., Slonim, D.K., Tamayo, P., Huard, C., Gaasenbeek, M., Mesirov, J.P., Coller, H., Loh, M.L., Downing, J.R., Caligiuri, M.A. *et al.* (1999) Molecular classification of cancer: class discovery and class prediction by gene expression monitoring. *Science*, **286**, 531-7.
228. Alizadeh, A.A., Eisen, M.B., Davis, R.E., Ma, C., Lossos, I.S., Rosenwald, A., Boldrick, J.C., Sabet, H., Tran, T., Yu, X. *et al.* (2000) Distinct types of diffuse large B-cell lymphoma identified by gene expression profiling. *Nature*, **403**, 503-11.
229. van 't Veer, L.J., Dai, H., van de Vijver, M.J., He, Y.D., Hart, A.A., Mao, M., Peterse, H.L., van der Kooy, K., Marton, M.J., Witteveen, A.T. *et al.* (2002) Gene expression profiling predicts clinical outcome of breast cancer. *Nature*, **415**, 530-6.
230. Huang, E., Cheng, S.H., Dressman, H., Pittman, J., Tsou, M.H., Horng, C.F., Bild, A., Iversen, E.S., Liao, M., Chen, C.M. *et al.* (2003) Gene expression predictors of breast cancer outcomes. *Lancet*, **361**, 1590-6.
231. Bittner, M., Meltzer, P., Chen, Y., Jiang, Y., Seftor, E., Hendrix, M., Radmacher, M., Simon, R., Yakhini, Z., Ben-Dor, A. *et al.* (2000) Molecular classification of cutaneous malignant melanoma by gene expression profiling. *Nature*, **406**, 536-40.
232. Whitfield, M.L., Finlay, D.R., Murray, J.I., Troyanskaya, O.G., Chi, J.T., Pergamenschikov, A., McCalmont, T.H., Brown, P.O., Botstein, D. and Connolly, M.K. (2003) Systemic and cell type-specific gene expression patterns in scleroderma skin. *Proc Natl Acad Sci U S A*, **100**, 12319-24.
233. Bowcock, A.M., Shannon, W., Du, F., Duncan, J., Cao, K., Aftergut, K., Catier, J., Fernandez-Vina, M.A. and Menter, A. (2001) Insights into psoriasis and other inflammatory diseases from large-scale gene expression studies. *Hum Mol Genet*, **10**, 1793-805.
234. Kim, C.J., Reintgen, D.S. and Yeatman, T.J. (2002) The promise of microarray technology in melanoma care. *Cancer Control*, **9**, 49-53.
235. DeRisi, J., Penland, L., Brown, P.O., Bittner, M.L., Meltzer, P.S., Ray, M., Chen, Y., Su, Y.A. and Trent, J.M. (1996) Use of a cDNA microarray to analyse gene expression patterns in human cancer. *Nat Genet*, **14**, 457-60.
236. Clark, E.A., Golub, T.R., Lander, E.S. and Hynes, R.O. (2000) Genomic analysis of metastasis reveals an essential role for RhoC. *Nature*, **406**, 532-5.
237. Carr, K.M., Bittner, M. and Trent, J.M. (2003) Gene-expression profiling in human cutaneous melanoma. *Oncogene*, **22**, 3076-80.
238. Haqq, C., Nosrati, M., Sudilovsky, D., Crothers, J., Khodabakhsh, D., Pulliam, B.L., Federman, S., Miller, J.R., 3rd, Allen, R.E., Singer, M.I. *et al.* (2005) The gene expression signatures of melanoma progression. *Proc Natl Acad Sci U S A*, **102**, 6092-7.
239. McGill, G.G., Horstmann, M., Widlund, H.R., Du, J., Motykova, G., Nishimura, E.K., Lin, Y.L., Ramaswamy, S., Avery, W., Ding, H.F. *et al.* (2002) Bcl2 regulation by the melanocyte master regulator Mitf modulates lineage survival and melanoma cell viability. *Cell*, **109**, 707-18.
240. Seftor, R.E., Seftor, E.A., Koshikawa, N., Meltzer, P.S., Gardner, L.M., Bilban, M., Stetler-Stevenson, W.G., Quaranta, V. and Hendrix, M.J. (2001) Cooperative interactions of laminin 5 gamma2 chain, matrix metalloproteinase-2, and membrane type-1-

matrix/metalloproteinase are required for mimicry of embryonic vasculogenesis by aggressive melanoma. *Cancer Res,* **61,** 6322-7.
241. Pavey, S., Johansson, P., Packer, L., Taylor, J., Stark, M., Pollock, P.M., Walker, G.J., Boyle, G.M., Harper, U., Cozzi, S.J. *et al.* (2004) Microarray expression profiling in melanoma reveals a BRAF mutation signature. *Oncogene,* **23,** 4060-7.
242. Tanami, H., Imoto, I., Hirasawa, A., Yuki, Y., Sonoda, I., Inoue, J., Yasui, K., Misawa-Furihata, A., Kawakami, Y. and Inazawa, J. (2004) Involvement of overexpressed wild-type BRAF in the growth of malignant melanoma cell lines. *Oncogene,* **23,** 8796-804.
243. Yuen, S.T., Davies, H., Chan, T.L., Ho, J.W., Bignell, G.R., Cox, C., Stephens, P., Edkins, S., Tsui, W.W., Chan, A.S. *et al.* (2002) Similarity of the phenotypic patterns associated with BRAF and KRAS mutations in colorectal neoplasia. *Cancer Res,* **62,** 6451-5.
244. Kumar, R., Angelini, S., Czene, K., Sauroja, I., Hahka-Kemppinen, M., Pyrhonen, S. and Hemminki, K. (2003) BRAF mutations in metastatic melanoma: a possible association with clinical outcome. *Clin Cancer Res,* **9,** 3362-8.
245. Singer, G., Oldt, R., 3rd, Cohen, Y., Wang, B.G., Sidransky, D., Kurman, R.J. and Shih Ie, M. (2003) Mutations in BRAF and KRAS characterize the development of low-grade ovarian serous carcinoma. *J Natl Cancer Inst,* **95,** 484-6.
246. Papp, T., Pemsel, H., Rollwitz, I., Schipper, H., Weiss, D.G., Schiffmann, D. and Zimmermann, R. (2003) Mutational analysis of N-ras, p53, CDKN2A (p16(INK4a)), p14(ARF), CDK4, and MC1R genes in human dysplastic melanocytic naevi. *J Med Genet,* **40,** E14.
247. Wang, H., Presland, R.B. and Piepkorn, M. (2005) A search for CDKN2A/p16INK4a mutations in melanocytic nevi from patients with melanoma and spouse controls by use of laser-captured microdissection. *Arch Dermatol,* **141,** 177-80.
248. Naldi, L., Lorenzo Imberti, G., Parazzini, F., Gallus, S. and La Vecchia, C. (2000) Pigmentary traits, modalities of sun reaction, history of sunburns, and melanocytic nevi as risk factors for cutaneous malignant melanoma in the Italian population: results of a collaborative case-control study. *Cancer,* **88,** 2703-10.
249. Harrison, S.L., MacKie, R.M. and MacLennan, R. (2000) Development of melanocytic nevi in the first three years of life. *J Natl Cancer Inst,* **92,** 1436-8.
250. Maldonado, J.L., Fridlyand, J., Patel, H., Jain, A.N., Busam, K., Kageshita, T., Ono, T., Albertson, D.G., Pinkel, D. and Bastian, B.C. (2003) Determinants of BRAF mutations in primary melanomas. *J Natl Cancer Inst,* **95,** 1878-90.
251. Van der Lubbe, J.L., Rosdorff, H.J., Bos, J.L. and Van der Eb, A.J. (1988) Activation of N-ras induced by ultraviolet irradiation in vitro. *Oncogene Res,* **3,** 9-20.
252. Winnepenninckx, V. and van den Oord, J.J. (2004) p16INK4A expression in malignant melanomas with or without a contiguous naevus remnant: a clue to their divergent pathogenesis? *Melanoma Res,* **14,** 321-2.
253. Kannan, K., Sharpless, N.E., Xu, J., O'Hagan, R.C., Bosenberg, M. and Chin, L. (2003) Components of the Rb pathway are critical targets of UV mutagenesis in a murine melanoma model. *Proc Natl Acad Sci U S A,* **100,** 1221-5.
254. Recio, J.A., Noonan, F.P., Takayama, H., Anver, M.R., Duray, P., Rush, W.L., Lindner, G., De Fabo, E.C., DePinho, R.A. and Merlino, G. (2002) Ink4a/arf deficiency promotes ultraviolet radiation-induced melanomagenesis. *Cancer Res,* **62,** 6724-30.
255. Hoa, M., Davis, S.L., Ames, S.J. and Spanjaard, R.A. (2002) Amplification of wild-type K-ras promotes growth of head and neck squamous cell carcinoma. *Cancer Res,* **62,** 7154-6.
256. Hingorani, S.R., Jacobetz, M.A., Robertson, G.P., Herlyn, M. and Tuveson, D.A. (2003) Suppression of BRAF(V599E) in human melanoma abrogates transformation. *Cancer Res,* **63,** 5198-202.
257. Calipel, A., Lefevre, G., Pouponnot, C., Mouriaux, F., Eychene, A. and Mascarelli, F. (2003) Mutation of B-Raf in human choroidal melanoma cells mediates cell proliferation and transformation through the MEK/ERK pathway. *J Biol Chem,* **278,** 42409-18.

258. Ohtani, N., Zebedee, Z., Huot, T.J., Stinson, J.A., Sugimoto, M., Ohashi, Y., Sharrocks, A.D., Peters, G. and Hara, E. (2001) Opposing effects of Ets and Id proteins on p16INK4a expression during cellular senescence. *Nature,* **409,** 1067-70.
259. Ikawa, S., Fukui, M., Ueyama, Y., Tamaoki, N., Yamamoto, T. and Toyoshima, K. (1988) B-raf, a new member of the raf family, is activated by DNA rearrangement. *Mol Cell Biol,* **8,** 2651-4.
260. Miki, T., Fleming, T.P., Crescenzi, M., Molloy, C.J., Blam, S.B., Reynolds, S.H. and Aaronson, S.A. (1991) Development of a highly efficient expression cDNA cloning system: application to oncogene isolation. *Proc Natl Acad Sci U S A,* **88,** 5167-71.
261. Furukawa, T., Sunamura, M., Motoi, F., Matsuno, S. and Horii, A. (2003) Potential tumor suppressive pathway involving DUSP6/MKP-3 in pancreatic cancer. *Am J Pathol,* **162,** 1807-15.
262. Hanafusa, H., Torii, S., Yasunaga, T. and Nishida, E. (2002) Sprouty1 and Sprouty2 provide a control mechanism for the Ras/MAPK signalling pathway. *Nat Cell Biol,* **4,** 850-8.
263. Kanai, F., Marignani, P.A., Sarbassova, D., Yagi, R., Hall, R.A., Donowitz, M., Hisaminato, A., Fujiwara, T., Ito, Y., Cantley, L.C. *et al.* (2000) TAZ: a novel transcriptional co-activator regulated by interactions with 14-3-3 and PDZ domain proteins. *Embo J,* **19,** 6778-91.
264. Stahl, J.M., Sharma, A., Cheung, M., Zimmerman, M., Cheng, J.Q., Bosenberg, M.W., Kester, M., Sandirasegarane, L. and Robertson, G.P. (2004) Deregulated Akt3 activity promotes development of malignant melanoma. *Cancer Res,* **64,** 7002-10.
265. Theodosiou, A. and Ashworth, A. (2002) MAP kinase phosphatases. *Genome Biol,* **3,** REVIEWS3009.
266. Dougherty, M.K., Muller, J., Ritt, D.A., Zhou, M., Zhou, X.Z., Copeland, T.D., Conrads, T.P., Veenstra, T.D., Lu, K.P. and Morrison, D.K. (2005) Regulation of Raf-1 by direct feedback phosphorylation. *Mol Cell,* **17,** 215-24.
267. Tsavachidou, D., Coleman, M.L., Athanasiadis, G., Li, S., Licht, J.D., Olson, M.F. and Weber, B.L. (2004) SPRY2 is an inhibitor of the ras/extracellular signal-regulated kinase pathway in melanocytes and melanoma cells with wild-type BRAF but not with the V599E mutant. *Cancer Res,* **64,** 5556-9.
268. Yusoff, P., Lao, D.H., Ong, S.H., Wong, E.S., Lim, J., Lo, T.L., Leong, H.F., Fong, C.W. and Guy, G.R. (2002) Sprouty2 inhibits the Ras/MAP kinase pathway by inhibiting the activation of Raf. *J Biol Chem,* **277,** 3195-201.
269. Palacios, E.H. and Weiss, A. (2004) Function of the Src-family kinases, Lck and Fyn, in T-cell development and activation. *Oncogene,* **23,** 7990-8000.
270. Iida, J., Wilhelmson, K.L., Price, M.A., Wilson, C.M., Pei, D., Furcht, L.T. and McCarthy, J.B. (2004) Membrane type-1 matrix metalloproteinase promotes human melanoma invasion and growth. *J Invest Dermatol,* **122,** 167-76.
271. Oikawa, T. (2004) ETS transcription factors: possible targets for cancer therapy. *Cancer Sci,* **95,** 626-33.
272. Giese, T., Engstner, M., Mansmann, U., Hartschuh, W. and Arden, B. (2005) Quantification of melanoma micrometastases in sentinel lymph nodes using real-time RT-PCR. *J Invest Dermatol,* **124,** 633-7.
273. Takeuchi, H., Morton, D.L., Kuo, C., Turner, R.R., Elashoff, D., Elashoff, R., Taback, B., Fujimoto, A. and Hoon, D.S. (2004) Prognostic significance of molecular upstaging of paraffin-embedded sentinel lymph nodes in melanoma patients. *J Clin Oncol,* **22,** 2671-80.
274. Bostick, P.J., Morton, D.L., Turner, R.R., Huynh, K.T., Wang, H.J., Elashoff, R., Essner, R. and Hoon, D.S. (1999) Prognostic significance of occult metastases detected by sentinel lymphadenectomy and reverse transcriptase-polymerase chain reaction in early-stage melanoma patients. *J Clin Oncol,* **17,** 3238-44.
275. Nagai, H., Hara, I., Horikawa, T., Oka, M., Kamidono, S. and Ichihashi, M. (2002) Gene transfer of secreted-type modified interleukin-18 gene to B16F10 melanoma cells suppresses

in vivo tumor growth through inhibition of tumor vessel formation. *J Invest Dermatol,* **119**, 541-8.
276. Kristiansen, G., Sammar, M. and Altevogt, P. (2004) Tumour biological aspects of CD24, a mucin-like adhesion molecule. *J Mol Histol,* **35**, 255-62.
277. Bieker, J.J. (2001) Kruppel-like factors: three fingers in many pies. *J Biol Chem,* **276**, 34355-8.
278. Russell, R.G., Lasorella, A., Dettin, L.E. and Iavarone, A. (2004) Id2 drives differentiation and suppresses tumor formation in the intestinal epithelium. *Cancer Res,* **64**, 7220-5.
279. Curtin, J.A., Fridlyand, J., Kageshita, T., Patel, H.N., Busam, K.J., Kutzner, H., Cho, K.H., Aiba, S., Brocker, E.B., LeBoit, P.E. et al. (2005) Distinct sets of genetic alterations in melanoma. *N Engl J Med,* **353**, 2135-47.
280. Clark, P.A., Llanos, S. and Peters, G. (2002) Multiple interacting domains contribute to p14ARF mediated inhibition of MDM2. *Oncogene,* **21**, 4498-507.
281. Berggren, P., Kumar, R., Sakano, S., Hemminki, L., Wada, T., Steineck, G., Adolfsson, J., Larsson, P., Norming, U., Wijkstrom, H. et al. (2003) Detecting homozygous deletions in the CDKN2A(p16(INK4a))/ARF(p14(ARF)) gene in urinary bladder cancer using real-time quantitative PCR. *Clin Cancer Res,* **9**, 235-42.
282. Sugumaran, M. (2002) Comparative biochemistry of eumelanogenesis and the protective roles of phenoloxidase and melanin in insects. *Pigment Cell Res,* **15**, 2-9.
283. Yasumoto, K., Takeda, K., Saito, H., Watanabe, K., Takahashi, K. and Shibahara, S. (2002) Microphthalmia-associated transcription factor interacts with LEF-1, a mediator of Wnt signaling. *Embo J,* **21**, 2703-14.
284. Loercher, A.E., Tank, E.M., Delston, R.B. and Harbour, J.W. (2005) MITF links differentiation with cell cycle arrest in melanocytes by transcriptional activation of INK4A. *J Cell Biol,* **168**, 35-40.
285. Zhang, H., Kobayashi, R., Galaktionov, K. and Beach, D. (1995) p19Skp1 and p45Skp2 are essential elements of the cyclin A-CDK2 S phase kinase. *Cell,* **82**, 915-25.
286. Nickoloff, B.J., Chaturvedi, V., Bacon, P., Qin, J.Z., Denning, M.F. and Diaz, M.O. (2000) Id-1 delays senescence but does not immortalize keratinocytes. *J Biol Chem,* **275**, 27501-4.
287. Zendman, A.J., Ruiter, D.J. and Van Muijen, G.N. (2003) Cancer/testis-associated genes: identification, expression profile, and putative function. *J Cell Physiol,* **194**, 272-88.
288. Furuta, J., Umebayashi, Y., Miyamoto, K., Kikuchi, K., Otsuka, F., Sugimura, T. and Ushijima, T. (2004) Promoter methylation profiling of 30 genes in human malignant melanoma. *Cancer Sci,* **95**, 962-8.
289. Eichmuller, S., Usener, D., Jochim, A. and Schadendorf, D. (2002) mRNA expression of tumor-associated antigens in melanoma tissues and cell lines. *Exp Dermatol,* **11**, 292-301.
290. Seykora, J.T., Jih, D., Elenitsas, R., Horng, W.H. and Elder, D.E. (2003) Gene expression profiling of melanocytic lesions. *Am J Dermatopathol,* **25**, 6-11.
291. Ribatti, D., Vacca, A., Ria, R., Marzullo, A., Nico, B., Filotico, R., Roncali, L. and Dammacco, F. (2003) Neovascularisation, expression of fibroblast growth factor-2, and mast cells with tryptase activity increase simultaneously with pathological progression in human malignant melanoma. *Eur J Cancer,* **39**, 666-74.
292. Birck, A., Kirkin, A.F., Zeuthen, J. and Hou-Jensen, K. (1999) Expression of basic fibroblast growth factor and vascular endothelial growth factor in primary and metastatic melanoma from the same patients. *Melanoma Res,* **9**, 375-81.
293. Alanko, T., Rosenberg, M. and Saksela, O. (1999) FGF expression allows nevus cells to survive in three-dimensional collagen gel under conditions that induce apoptosis in normal human melanocytes. *J Invest Dermatol,* **113**, 111-6.
294. Marin, Y.E., Namkoong, J., Cohen-Solal, K., Shin, S.S., Martino, J.J., Oka, M. and Chen, S. (2005) Stimulation of oncogenic metabotropic glutamate receptor 1 in melanoma cells activates ERK1/2 via PKCepsilon. *Cell Signal.*

295. Pollock, P.M., Cohen-Solal, K., Sood, R., Namkoong, J., Martino, J.J., Koganti, A., Zhu, H., Robbins, C., Makalowska, I., Shin, S.S. *et al.* (2003) Melanoma mouse model implicates metabotropic glutamate signaling in melanocytic neoplasia. *Nat Genet,* **34,** 108-12.
296. Cavalheiro, E.A. and Olney, J.W. (2001) Glutamate antagonists: deadly liaisons with cancer. *Proc Natl Acad Sci U S A,* **98,** 5947-8.
297. Oda, K., Arakawa, H., Tanaka, T., Matsuda, K., Tanikawa, C., Mori, T., Nishimori, H., Tamai, K., Tokino, T., Nakamura, Y. *et al.* (2000) p53AIP1, a potential mediator of p53-dependent apoptosis, and its regulation by Ser-46-phosphorylated p53. *Cell,* **102,** 849-62.
298. Marsters, S.A., Sheridan, J.P., Donahue, C.J., Pitti, R.M., Gray, C.L., Goddard, A.D., Bauer, K.D. and Ashkenazi, A. (1996) Apo-3, a new member of the tumor necrosis factor receptor family, contains a death domain and activates apoptosis and NF-kappa B. *Curr Biol,* **6,** 1669-76.
299. Gutgemann, A., Golob, M., Muller, S., Buettner, R. and Bosserhoff, A.K. (2001) Isolation of invasion-associated cDNAs in melanoma. *Arch Dermatol Res,* **293,** 283-90.
300. Luo, B., Aster, J.C., Hasserjian, R.P., Kuo, F. and Sklar, J. (1997) Isolation and functional analysis of a cDNA for human Jagged2, a gene encoding a ligand for the Notch1 receptor. *Mol Cell Biol,* **17,** 6057-67.
301. Lanford, P.J., Lan, Y., Jiang, R., Lindsell, C., Weinmaster, G., Gridley, T. and Kelley, M.W. (1999) Notch signalling pathway mediates hair cell development in mammalian cochlea. *Nat Genet,* **21,** 289-92.
302. Artavanis-Tsakonas, S., Rand, M.D. and Lake, R.J. (1999) Notch signaling: cell fate control and signal integration in development. *Science,* **284,** 770-6.
303. Cereseto, A. and Tsai, S. (2000) Jagged2 induces cell cycling in confluent fibroblasts susceptible to density-dependent inhibition of cell division. *J Cell Physiol,* **185,** 425-31.

8. APPENDIX

Table 9. List and classification of genes upregulated in melanoma cell lines with the *B-RAF* and/or *N-RAS* mutations obtained from the analysis of microarray data with 3 different softwares.

Molecular Function / Gene Title	Gene Symbol	Fold Change
A. Genes overexpressed in cell lines with *B-RAF* and *N-RAS* mutations		
Signal Transducer Activity		
SH3 domain binding glutamic acid-rich protein like	SH3BGRL	213
Transporter Activity		
solute carrier family 2 (facilitated glucose transporter), member 3	SLC2A3	56
Catalytic Activity		
dual specificity phosphatase 6	DUSP6	13
peroxisomal D3,D2-enoyl-CoA isomerase	PECI	211
tribbles homolog 2 (Drosophila)	TRIB2	42
v-akt murine thymoma viral oncogene homolog 3 (protein kinase B, gamma)	AKT3	7
vesicle amine transport protein 1 homolog (T californica)	VAT1	8
Binding Activity		
peroxisomal D3,D2-enoyl-CoA isomerase	PECI	211
tribbles homolog 2 (Drosophila)	TRIB2	42
v-akt murine thymoma viral oncogene homolog 3 (protein kinase B, gamma)	AKT3	7
vesicle amine transport protein 1 homolog (T californica)	VAT1	8
vimentin	VIM	155
Structural Molecule Activity		
vimentin	VIM	155
No Classification		
armadillo repeat containing, X-linked 1	ARMCX1	7
DnaJ (Hsp40) homolog, subfamily D, member 1	DNAJD1	127
HOM-TES-103 tumor antigen-like	HOM-TES-103	8
B. Genes overexpressed in cell lines with *B-RAF* mutation		
Signal Transducer Activity		
HMT1 hnRNP methyltransferase-like 1 (S. cerevisiae)	HRMT1L1	4
lectin, galactoside-binding, soluble, 1 (galectin 1)	LGALS1	10
lymphocyte antigen 96	LY96	41
pre-B-cell colony enhancing factor 1	PBEF1	4
Binding Activity		
Branched chain alpha-ketoacid dehydrogenase kinase	BCKDK	3
cartilage paired-class homeoprotein 1	CART1	51
dishevelled associated activator of morphogenesis 2	DAAM2	6
FYN oncogene related to SRC, FGR, YES	FYN	7
lectin, galactoside-binding, soluble, 1 (galectin 1)	LGALS1	10
matrix metalloproteinase 14 (membrane-inserted)	MMP14	10
mitochondrial folate transporter/carrier	MFTC	4

pre-B-cell colony enhancing factor 1	PBEF1	4
Rhomboid family 1 (Drosophila)	RHBDF1	4
sarcoglycan, epsilon	SGCE	90
secreted protein, acidic, cysteine-rich (osteonectin)	SPARC	290
serine (or cysteine) proteinase inhibitor, clade E (nexin, plasminogen activator inhibitor type 1), member 2	SERPINE2	6
sushi-repeat-containing protein, X-linked	SRPX	43
transcriptional co-activator with PDZ-binding motif (TAZ)	TAZ	5
valyl-tRNA synthetase 2	VARS2	4
Transcription Regulator Activity		
cartilage paired-class homeoprotein 1	CART1	51
transcriptional co-activator with PDZ-binding motif (TAZ)	TAZ	5
Catalytic Activity		
Branched chain alpha-ketoacid dehydrogenase kinase	BCKDK	3
FYN oncogene related to SRC, FGR, YES	FYN	7
HMT1 hnRNP methyltransferase-like 1 (S. cerevisiae)	HRMT1L1	4
matrix metalloproteinase 14 (membrane-inserted)	MMP14	10
nudix (nucleoside diphosphate linked moiety X)-type motif 3	NUDT3	3
pre-B-cell colony enhancing factor 1	PBEF1	4
protein phosphatase 1, regulatory (inhibitor) subunit 3C	PPP1R3C	10
valyl-tRNA synthetase 2	VARS2	4
Enzyme Regulator Activity		
serine (or cysteine) proteinase inhibitor, clade E (nexin, plasminogen activator inhibitor type 1), member 2	SERPINE2	6
sprouty homolog 2 (Drosophila)	SPRY2	15
Transporter Activity		
mitochondrial folate transporter/carrier	MFTC	4
solute carrier family 2 (facilitated glucose transporter), member 14	SLC2A14	26
solute carrier family 29 (nucleoside transporters), member 1	SLC29A1	6
No Classification		
chromosome 6 open reading frame 11	C6orf11	7
melanoma antigen, family A, 3	MAGEA3	111
melanoma antigen, family D, 2	MAGED2	4
peripheral myelin protein 22	PMP22	22
popeye domain containing 3	POPDC3	11
suppression of tumorigenicity	ST7	14
taxol resistance associated gene 3	TRAG3	115
<u>C. Genes overexpressed in cell lines with *N-RAS* mutation</u>		
Structural Molecule Activity		
actin related protein 2/3 complex, subunit 1B, 41kDa	ARPC1B	5
Transcription Regulator Activity		
Cbp/p300-interacting transactivator, with Glu/Asp-rich carboxy-terminal domain, 1	CITED1	51
ets variant gene 4 (E1A enhancer binding protein, E1AF)	ETV4	9
ets variant gene 5 (ets-related molecule)	ETV5	13
leucine zipper, putative tumor suppressor 1	LZTS1	28
MADS box transcription enhancer factor 2, polypeptide C	MEF2C	21

Neuronal PAS domain protein 2	NPAS2	7
SRY (sex determining region Y)-box 10	SOX10	50
zinc finger homeobox 1b	ZFHX1B	53
Signal Transducer Activity		
amyotrophic lateral sclerosis 2 (juvenile) chromosome region, candidate 3	ALS2CR3	4
ATPase, H+ transporting, lysosomal 42kDa, V1 subunit C, isoform 1	ATP6V1C1	3
Discoidin domain receptor family, member 2	DDR2	27
endothelin receptor type B	EDNRB	231
G protein-coupled receptor 143	GPR143	61
G protein-coupled receptor 19	GPR19	21
Neuronal PAS domain protein 2	NPAS2	7
neuropilin 2	NRP2	4
Syndecan binding protein (syntenin)	SDCBP	3
TNF receptor-associated factor 5	TRAF5	9
transient receptor potential cation channel, subfamily V, member 2	TRPV2	15
tumor necrosis factor receptor superfamily, member 14 (herpesvirus entry mediator)	TNFRSF14	37
type I transmembrane C-type lectin receptor DCL-1	DCL-1	54
Binding Activity		
acyl-CoA synthetase long-chain family member 3	ACSL3	3
adaptor-related protein complex 1, sigma 2 subunit	AP1S2	12
amyotrophic lateral sclerosis 2 (juvenile) chromosome region, candidate 3	ALS2CR3	4
ATPase, H+ transporting, lysosomal 42kDa, V1 subunit C, isoform 1	ATP6V1C1	3
ATPase, H+ transporting, lysosomal 56/58kDa, V1 subunit B, isoform 2	ATP6V1B2	4
baculoviral IAP repeat-containing 7 (livin)	BIRC7	18
Cbp/p300-interacting transactivator, with Glu/Asp-rich carboxy-terminal domain, 1	CITED1	51
Discoidin domain receptor family, member 2	DDR2	27
dopachrome tautomerase (dopachrome delta-isomerase, tyrosine-related protein 2)	DCT	92
endothelin receptor type B	EDNRB	231
ets variant gene 4 (E1A enhancer binding protein, E1AF)	ETV4	9
ets variant gene 5 (ets-related molecule)	ETV5	13
Influenza virus NS1A binding protein	IVNS1ABP	4
leucine zipper, putative tumor suppressor 1	LZTS1	28
MADS box transcription enhancer factor 2, polypeptide C (myocyte enhancer factor 2C)	MEF2C	21
Neuronal PAS domain protein 2	NPAS2	7
parvin, beta	PARVB	27
PDZ domain containing RING finger 3	PDZRN3	136
quaking homolog, KH domain RNA binding (mouse)	QKI	11
ras homolog gene family, member Q	RHOQ	10
SRY (sex determining region Y)-box 10	SOX10	50
Syndecan binding protein (syntenin)	SDCBP	3
TNF receptor-associated factor 5	TRAF5	9
tumor necrosis factor receptor superfamily, member 14 (herpesvirus entry mediator)	TNFRSF14	37
type I transmembrane C-type lectin receptor DCL-1	DCL-1	54
WAS protein family, member 3	WASF3	5
zinc finger homeobox 1b	ZFHX1B	53
zinc finger protein 238	ZNF238	4
zinc finger protein 330	ZNF330	3

Catalytic Activity		
Acetyl-Coenzyme A acyltransferase 2		
acyl-CoA synthetase long-chain family member 3	ACSL3	3
ATPase, H+ transporting, lysosomal 42kDa, V1 subunit C, isoform 1	ATP6V1C1	3
ATPase, H+ transporting, lysosomal 56/58kDa, V1 subunit B, isoform 2	ATP6V1B2	4
baculoviral IAP repeat-containing 7 (livin)	BIRC7	18
cytochrome P450, family 27, subfamily A, polypeptide 1	CYP27A1	19
Discoidin domain receptor family, member 2	DDR2	27
dopachrome tautomerase (dopachrome delta-isomerase, tyrosine-related protein 2)	DCT	92
dual specificity phosphatase 4	DUSP4	11
glutathione S-transferase M1	GSTM1	4
glutathione S-transferase M4	GSTM4	32
hyaluronan synthase 2	HAS2	46
methionine sulfoxide reductase A	MSRA	3
N-acylsphingosine amidohydrolase (acid ceramidase) 1	ASAH1	7
neuropilin 2	NRP2	4
PDZ domain containing RING finger 3	PDZRN3	136
plasma glutamate carboxypeptidase	PGCP	37
polymerase (RNA) III (DNA directed) polypeptide G (32kD)	POLR3G	11
quinoid dihydropteridine reductase	QDPR	4
ras homolog gene family, member Q	RHOQ	10
sialyltransferase 9 (CMP-NeuAc:lactosylceramide alpha-2,3-sialyltransferase; GM3 synthase)	SIAT9	6
TNF receptor-associated factor 5	TRAF5	9
tyrosinase (oculocutaneous albinism IA)	TYR	84
Transporter Activity		
adaptor-related protein complex 1, sigma 2 subunit	AP1S2	12
amyotrophic lateral sclerosis 2 (juvenile) chromosome region, candidate 3	ALS2CR3	4
ATPase, H+ transporting, lysosomal 42kDa, V1 subunit C, isoform 1	ATP6V1C1	3
ATPase, H+ transporting, lysosomal 56/58kDa, V1 subunit B, isoform 2	ATP6V1B2	4
gap junction protein, beta 1, 32kDa (connexin 32, Charcot-Marie-Tooth neuropathy, X-linked)	GJB1	28
neuropilin 2	NRP2	4
quinoid dihydropteridine reductase	QDPR	4
six transmembrane epithelial antigen of the prostate	STEAP	4
solute carrier family 16 (monocarboxylic acid transporters), member 4	SLC16A4	227
transient receptor potential cation channel, subfamily V, member 2	TRPV2	15
Enzyme Regulator Activity		
zinc finger homeobox 1b	ZFHX1B	53
Motor Activity		
dynein, cytoplasmic, intermediate polypeptide 1	DNCI1	10
No Classification		
chromosome 9 open reading frame 91	C9orf91	3
epidermodysplasia verruciformis 1	EVER1	5
Epithelial membrane protein 3	EMP3	43
hypothetical protein LOC151162	LOC151162	8
junctional adhesion molecule 3	JAM3	6
lymphocyte adaptor protein	LNK	7
male sterility domain containing 1	MLSTD1	145
melan-A	MLANA	349

Melanophilin	MLPH	14
phosphatidylinositol glycan, class F	PIGF	208
Pleckstrin homology-like domain, family A, member 1	PHLDA1	5
preferentially expressed antigen in melanoma	PRAME	123
Ras-related GTP binding D	RRAGD	10
ring finger protein 144	RNF144	34
serologically defined colon cancer antigen 8	SDCCAG8	32
Synuclein, alpha (non A4 component of amyloid precursor)	SNCA	15
TCF3 (E2A) fusion partner (in childhood Leukemia)	TFPT	5
ubiquitin-like 3	UBL3	6
zinc finger, FYVE domain containing 16	ZFYVE16	4

Table 10. List and Classification of genes downregulated in melanoma cell lines with the *B-RAF* and/or *N-RAS* mutations obtained from the analysis of microarray data with 3 different softwares.

Molecular Function / Gene Name	Gene Symbol	Fold Change
A. Genes downregulated in cell lines with *B-RAF* and *N-RAS* mutations		
Catalytic Activity		
adenosine kinase	ADK	5
Annexin A3	ANXA3	97
argininosuccinate synthetase	ASS	101
chromosome 9 open reading frame 3	C9orf3	6
GTP cyclohydrolase 1 (dopa-responsive dystonia)	GCH1	5
macrophage stimulating 1 receptor (c-met-related tyrosine kinase)	MST1R	7
MCM2 minichromosome maintenance deficient 2, mitotin (S. cerevisiae)	MCM2	4
protein kinase C, iota	PRKCI	4
pyrophosphatase (inorganic)	PP	3
serine hydroxymethyltransferase 1 (soluble)	SHMT1	6
steroid-5-alpha-reductase, alpha polypeptide 1	SRD5A1	6
Structural Molecule Activity		
collagen, type IV, alpha 5 (Alport syndrome)	COL4A5	24
keratin 17	KRT17	73
keratin 18	KRT18	16
keratin 8	KRT8	73
laminin, beta 3	LAMB3	17
periplakin	PPL	107
tuftelin 1	TUFT1	6
Motor Activity		
myosin VC	MYO5C	6
Signal Transducer Activity		
amphiregulin (schwannoma-derived growth factor)	AREG	46
coagulation factor III (thromboplastin, tissue factor)	F3	37
interleukin 18 (interferon-gamma-inducing factor)	IL18	227
macrophage stimulating 1 receptor (c-met-related tyrosine kinase)	MST1R	7
protein kinase C, iota	PRKCI	4
sema domain, immunoglobulin domain (Ig), short basic domain, secreted, (semaphorin) 3F	SEMA3F	4
Transcription Regulator Activity		
homeo box A9	HOXA9	41
Kruppel-like factor 4 (gut)	KLF4	13
Kruppel-like factor 5 (intestinal)	KLF5	69
Tripartite motif-containing 29	TRIM29	192
Enzyme Regulator Activity		
Annexin A3	ANXA3	97
serine protease inhibitor, Kunitz type, 2	SPINT2	142
Stratifin	SFN	33
Transporter Activity		
laminin, beta 3	LAMB3	17
solute carrier family 29 (nucleoside transporters), member 3	SLC29A3	7

steroid-5-alpha-reductase, alpha polypeptide 1	SRD5A1	6
No Classification		
CD24 antigen (small cell lung carcinoma cluster 4 antigen)	CD24	428
chromosome 19 open reading frame 21	C19orf21	7
DnaJ (Hsp40) homolog, subfamily C, member 9	DNAJC9	4
EPS8-like 2	EPS8L2	46
hypothetical protein FLJ14054	FLJ14054	36
Inhibitor of DNA binding 1, dominant negative helix-loop-helix protein	ID1	83
keratin 19	KRT19	11
neuroepithelial cell transforming gene 1	NET1	6
podocalyxin-like	PODXL	10
sema domain, immunoglobulin domain (Ig), short basic domain, secreted, (semaphorin) 3F	SEMA3F	4
tumor necrosis factor, alpha-induced protein 8	TNFAIP8	10
B. Genes downregulated in cell lines with *B-RAF* mutation		
Catalytic Activity		
abhydrolase domain containing 3	ABHD3	4
aldehyde dehydrogenase 3 family, member A2	ALDH3A2	4
amylo-1, 6-glucosidase, 4-alpha-glucanotransferase (glycogen debranching enzyme, glycogen storage disease type III)	AGL	4
F-box only protein 3	FBXO3	3
phosphatidic acid phosphatase type 2C	PPAP2C	3
phosphorylase kinase, beta	PHKB	3
phosphoserine phosphatase	PSPH	13
protein tyrosine phosphatase, receptor type, F	PTPRF	16
zinc finger, BED domain containing 1	ZBED1	3
Structural Molecule Activity		
fibulin 1	FBLN1	15
plakophilin 3	PKP3	8
Signal Transducer Activity		
diaphanous homolog 1 (Drosophila)	DIAPH1	4
protein tyrosine phosphatase, receptor type, F	PTPRF	16
Binding Activity		
actin binding LIM protein 1	ABLIM1	17
desmoglein 2	DSG2	17
diaphanous homolog 1 (Drosophila)	DIAPH1	4
erythrocyte membrane protein band 4.1 like 4B	EPB41L4B	7
fibulin 1	FBLN1	15
heterogeneous nuclear ribonucleoprotein H3 (2H9)	HNRPH3	4
LAG1 longevity assurance homolog 6 (S. cerevisiae)	LASS6	4
phosphorylase kinase, beta	PHKB	3
phosphoserine phosphatase	PSPH	13
plakophilin 3	PKP3	7
protein tyrosine phosphatase, receptor type, F	PTPRF	16
zinc finger, BED domain containing 1	ZBED1	3
Transcription Regulator Activity		
LAG1 longevity assurance homolog 6 (S. cerevisiae)	LASS6	4

Enzyme Regulator Activity		
phosphorylase kinase, beta	PHKB	3

Transporter Activity		
solute carrier family 38, member 1	SLC38A1	115
solute carrier family 7 (cationic amino acid transporter), member 5	SLC7A5	10

No Classification		
cordon-bleu homolog (mouse)	COBL	42
G protein-coupled receptor 48	GPR48	11
hypothetical protein FLJ22662	FLJ22662	13
hypothetical protein KIAA1164	KIAA1164	5
Inhibitor of DNA binding 2, dominant negative helix-loop-helix protein	ID2	6
KIAA0431 protein	KIAA0431	3
KIAA0746 protein	KIAA0746	8
neural proliferation, differentiation and control, 1	NPDC1	15
PERP, TP53 apoptosis effector	PERP	31
programmed cell death 4 (neoplastic transformation inhibitor)	PDCD4	9
Rab6-interacting protein 2	ELKS	4
transducin-like enhancer of split 2 (E(sp1) homolog, Drosophila)	TLE2	5
ubiquitously transcribed tetratricopeptide repeat, X chromosome	UTX	4

C. Genes downregulated in cell lines with *N-RAS* mutation

Catalytic Activity		
B cell RAG associated protein	GALNAC4S-6ST	31
carbohydrate (chondroitin 6) sulfotransferase 3	CHST3	5
EH-domain containing 2	EHD2	37
Hypoxia-inducible factor prolyl 4-hydroxylase	PH-4	9
polymerase (DNA directed) sigma	POLS	3
RAD1 homolog (S. pombe)	RAD1	3
ras homolog gene family, member D	RHOD	4

Structural Molecule Activity		
plastin 1 (I isoform)	PLS1	4
vinculin	VCL	5

Transcription Regulator Activity		
sine oculis homeobox homolog 2 (Drosophila)	SIX2	6
Tripartite motif-containing 16	TRIM16	5
zinc finger protein 131 (clone pHZ-10)	ZNF131	3

Motor Activity		
Ras interacting protein 1	RASIP1	28

Binding Activity		
Annexin A7	ANXA7	4
B cell RAG associated protein	GALNAC4S-6ST	31
Capping protein (actin filament), gelsolin-like	CAPG	9
dickkopf homolog 1 (Xenopus laevis)	DKK1	36
EH-domain containing 2	EHD2	37
heat shock 70kDa protein 1A	HSPA1A	4
heat shock 70kDa protein 1B	HSPA1B	3

Hypoxia-inducible factor prolyl 4-hydroxylase	PH-4	9
oxysterol binding protein-like 3	OSBPL3	4
plastin 1 (I isoform)	PLS1	4
poly(A) binding protein interacting protein 1	PAIP1	4
polymerase (DNA directed) sigma	POLS	3
RAD1 homolog (S. pombe)	RAD1	3
ras homolog gene family, member D	RHOD	4
related RAS viral (r-ras) oncogene homolog 2	RRAS2	4
ryanodine receptor 1 (skeletal)	RYR1	35
sine oculis homeobox homolog 2 (Drosophila)	SIX2	7
thymosin, beta 4, X-linked	TMSB4X	14
Tripartite motif-containing 16	TRIM16	5
vinculin	VCL	5
zinc finger protein 131 (clone pHZ-10)	ZNF131	4
Signal Transducer Activity		
adenosine A2b receptor	ADORA2B	15
dickkopf homolog 1 (Xenopus laevis)	DKK1	36
ryanodine receptor 1 (skeletal)	RYR1	35
secreted and transmembrane 1	SECTM1	36
Transporter Activity		
Annexin A7	ANXA7	4
ryanodine receptor 1 (skeletal)	RYR1	35
No Classification		
brain abundant, membrane attached signal protein 1	BASP1	150
golgi phosphoprotein 3 (coat-protein)	GOLPH3	4
growth arrest and DNA-damage-inducible, beta	GADD45B	3
hypothetical protein FLJ10233	FLJ10233	3
hypothetical protein FLJ20152	FLJ20152	5
hypothetical protein FLJ20364	FLJ20364	3
IDN3 protein	IDN3	5
KIAA0947 protein	KIAA0947	4
KIAA0974 mRNA	KIAA0974	4
polymerase I and transcript release factor	PTRF	30
RAN binding protein 6	RANBP6	3
RNA-binding protein	FLJ20273	14
testis derived transcript (3 LIM domains)	TES	3
trophoblast glycoprotein	TPBG	13

Table 11. List and Classification of genes overexpressed in melanoma cell lines with homozygous deletion of the *CDKN2A* gene obtained from analysis of microarray data with 3 different softwares.

Molecular Function/Gene Name	Gene Symbol	Fold Change* (95% CI)	P-value**
Structural Molecule Activity			
actin related protein 2/3 complex, subunit 1B, 41kDa	ARPC1B	4 (3.6 - 5.3)	0.015
extracellular matrix protein 1	ECM1	4 (3.5 - 4.8)	0.002
laminin, alpha 4	LAMA4	70 (33.3 - 106.6)	0.025
nestin	NES	34 (16.6 - 50.6)	0.010
vimentin	VIM	148 (119.9 - 176.0)	0.003
Transporter Activity			
adaptor-related protein complex 1, sigma 2 subunit	AP1S2	25 (14.2 - 35.7)	0.012
ATPase, H+ transporting, lysosomal 56/58kDa, V1 subunit B, isoform 2	ATP6V1B2	3 (2.8 - 4.2)	0.023
extracellular matrix protein 1	ECM1	4 (3.5 - 4.8)	0.002
solute carrier family 2 (facilitated glucose transporter), member 3	SLC2A3	67 (31.4 - 103.0)	0.003
solute carrier family 39 (zinc transporter), member 7	SLC39A7	4 (2.7 - 4.6)	0.007
Catalytic Activity			
acetyl-Coenzyme A acyltransferase 2	ACAA2	17 (8.0 - 25.7)	0.003
ATPase, H+ transporting, lysosomal 56/58kDa, V1 subunit B, isoform 2	ATP6V1B2	3 (2.8 - 4.2)	0.023
beta-site APP-cleaving enzyme 2	BACE2	14 (8.7 - 19.0)	0.003
calpain 3, (p94)	CAPN3	653 (448.1 - 858.7)	0.005
carbohydrate sulfotransferase 10	CHST10	3 (2.4 - 3.0)	0.009
cytochrome P450, family 27, subfamily A, polypeptide 1	CYP27A1	22 (17.8 - 26.5)	0.012
dopachrome tautomerase	DCT	42 (32.5 - 51.8)	0.001
dual specificity phosphatase 4	DUSP4	26 (13.9 - 38.6)	0.022
dual specificity phosphatase 6	DUSP6	67 (15.9 - 118.7)	0.012
F-box protein 7	FBXO7	3 (2.7 - 3.4)	0.001
FK506 binding protein 10, 65 kDa	FKBP10	59 (43.7 - 75.2)	0.012
N-acylsphingosine amidohydrolase (acid ceramidase) 1	ASAH1	3 (2.5 - 3.5)	0.013
peroxisomal D3,D2-enoyl-CoA isomerase	PECI	274 (120.7 -427.9)	0.025
phospholipase A1 member A	PLA1A	17 (10.1 - 23.8)	0.022
protein tyrosine phosphatase, receptor type, M	PTPRM	11 (8.4 - 13.7)	0.013
RAB38, member RAS oncogene family	RAB38	15 (4.5 - 25.0)	0.004
ras homolog gene family, member Q	RHOQ	17 (9.7 - 23.9)	0.013
sialyltransferase 4C (beta-galactoside alpha-2,3-sialyltransferase)	SIAT4C	5 (4.0 - 5.5)	0.002
sphingomyelin phosphodiesterase 1, acid lysosomal (acid sphingomyelinase)	SMPD1	3 (2.5 - 4.1)	0.000
tribbles homolog 2 (Drosophila)	TRIB2	10 (5.8 - 13.7)	0.013
tyrosinase (oculocutaneous albinism IA)	TYR	71 (45.7 - 96.6)	0.020
v-akt murine thymoma viral oncogene homolog 3 (protein kinase B, gamma)	AKT3	7 (4.8 - 8.3)	0.009
vesicle amine transport protein 1 homolog (T californica)	VAT1	8 (5.9 - 9.3)	0.013
Transcription Regulator Activity			
Down syndrome critical region gene 1	DSCR1	12 (8.3 - 15.4)	0.010
ets variant gene 5 (ets-related molecule)	ETV5	11 (7.9 - 14.7)	0.019
hairy/enhancer-of-split related with YRPW motif 1	HEY1	11 (6.8 - 14.3)	0.018
SRY (sex determining region Y)-box 10	SOX10	36 (30.8 - 41.9)	0.000

T-box 2	TBX2	36 (22.9 - 48.8)	0.015
Binding Activity			
adaptor-related protein complex 1, sigma 2 subunit	AP1S2	25 (14.2 - 35.7)	0.012
ATPase, H+ transporting, lysosomal 56/58kDa, V1 subunit B, isoform 2	ATP6V1B2	3 (2.8 - 4.2)	0.023
calpain 3, (p94)	CAPN3	653 (448.1 - 858.7)	0.005
deleted in liver cancer 1	DLC1	6 (3.8 - 8.3)	0.007
dopachrome tautomerase	DCT	42 (32.5 - 51.8)	0.001
Down syndrome critical region gene 1	DSCR1	12 (8.3 - 15.4)	0.010
endothelin receptor type B	EDNRB	105 (81.6 - 128.7)	0.004
ets variant gene 5 (ets-related molecule)	ETV5	11 (7.9 - 14.7)	0.019
FK506 binding protein 10, 65 kDa	FKBP10	59 (43.7 - 75.2)	0.012
gelsolin (amyloidosis, Finnish type)	GSN	5 (3.8 - 6.8)	0.003
hairy/enhancer-of-split related with YRPW motif 1	HEY1	11 (6.8 - 14.3)	0.018
integrin, beta 3 (platelet glycoprotein IIIa, antigen CD61)	ITGB3	28 (14.8 - 41.1)	0.000
laminin, alpha 4	LAMA4	70 (33.3 - 106.6)	0.025
leukemia inhibitory factor (cholinergic differentiation factor)	LIF	18 (11.3 - 23.7)	0.001
parvin, beta	PARVB	25 (15.4 - 35.1)	0.021
peroxisomal D3,D2-enoyl-CoA isomerase	PECI	274 (120.7 - 427.9)	0.025
protein kinase C binding protein 1	PRKCBP1	6 (3.5 - 8.3)	0.005
RAB38, member RAS oncogene family	RAB38	15 (4.5 - 25.0)	0.004
ras homolog gene family, member Q	RHOQ	17 (9.7 - 23.9)	0.013
secreted protein, acidic, cysteine-rich (osteonectin)	SPARC	383 (259.1 - 506.6)	0.016
serine (or cysteine) proteinase inhibitor, clade E, member 2	SERPINE2	11 (6.3 - 14.8)	0.003
SRY (sex determining region Y)-box 10	SOX10	36 (30.8 - 41.9)	0.000
T-box 2	TBX2	36 (22.9 - 48.8)	0.015
tribbles homolog 2 (Drosophila)	TRIB2	10 (5.8 - 13.7)	0.013
v-akt murine thymoma viral oncogene homolog 3 (protein kinase B, gamma)	AKT3	7 (4.8 - 8.3)	0.009
vesicle amine transport protein 1 homolog (T californica)	VAT1	8 (5.9 - 9.3)	0.013
vimentin	VIM	148 (119.9 - 176.0)	0.003
Signal Transducer Activity			
calpain 3, (p94)	CAPN3	653 (448.1 - 858.7)	0.005
CGI-141 protein	CGI-141	2 (2.1 - 2.6)	0.000
endothelin receptor type B	EDNRB	105 (81.6 - 128.7)	0.004
extracellular matrix protein 1	ECM1	4 (3.5 - 4.8)	0.002
integrin, beta 3 (platelet glycoprotein IIIa, antigen CD61)	ITGB3	28 (14.8 - 41.1)	0.000
laminin, alpha 4	LAMA4	70 (33.3 - 106.6)	0.025
leukemia inhibitory factor (cholinergic differentiation factor)	LIF	18 (11.3 - 23.7)	0.001
protein tyrosine phosphatase, receptor type, M	PTPRM	11 (8.4 - 13.7)	0.013
SH3 domain binding glutamic acid-rich protein like	SH3BGRL	517 (276.5 - 757.1)	0.008
No Classification			
chondroitin polymerizing factor	CHPF	3 (2.3 - 2.8)	0.007
chromosome 10 open reading frame 56	C10orf56	6 (4.5 - 7.7)	0.003
chromosome 16 open reading frame 23	C16orf23	6 (4.4 - 7.5)	0.022
CSAG family, member 2	CSAG2	227 (141.2 - 313.4)	0.017
epithelial membrane protein 3	EMP3	63 (32.4 - 94.1)	0.002
glycoprotein M6B	GPM6B	50 (35.7 - 63.4)	0.003
HOM-TES-103 tumor antigen-like	HOM-TES-103	8 (5.9 - 10.1)	0.002
hypothetical protein LOC151162	LOC151162	3 (2.4 - 4.3)	0.021
melanoma antigen, family A, 12	MAGEA12	90 (65.1 - 115.5)	0.001

melanoma antigen, family A, 2	MAGEA2	128 (82.8 - 172.2)	0.004
melanoma antigen, family A, 6	MAGEA6	623 (473.4 - 772.1)	0.001
osteopetrosis associated transmembrane protein 1	OSTM1	8 (5.1 - 11.6)	0.004
phosphatase and actin regulator 1	PHACTR1	114 (77.2 - 151.4)	0.006
popeye domain containing 3	POPDC3	12 (7.8 - 15.3)	0.009
proteolipid protein 1	PLP1	139 (97.7 - 179.5)	0.019
similar to Six transmembrane epithelial antigen of prostate	MGC87042	28 (20.3 - 34.7)	0.024
SNRPN upstream reading frame	SNURF	34 (7.8 - 60.3)	0.009
sorting nexin 10	SNX10	7 (4.4 - 8.8)	0.006
sprouty homolog 2 (Drosophila)	SPRY2	26 (15.1 - 36.5)	0.009
sprouty homolog 4 (Drosophila)	SPRY4	6 (4.5 - 7.4)	0.020
synuclein, alpha (non A4 component of amyloid precursor)	SNCA	30 (8.7 - 51.4)	0.014
TCF3 (E2A) fusion partner (in childhood Leukemia)	TFPT	5 (4.3 - 5.0)	0.000
transmembrane 7 superfamily member 1 (upregulated in kidney)	TM7SF1	9 (6.3 - 11.0)	0.005

Table 12. List and Classification of genes underexpressed in melanoma cell lines with homozygous deletion of *CDKN2A* gene obtained from analysis of microarray data with 3 different softwares.

Molecular Function/Gene Name	Gene Symbol	Fold Change* (95% CI)	P-value**
Signal Transducer Activity			
adenosine A2b receptor	ADORA2B	26 (6.0 - 45.1)	0.054
amphiregulin (schwannoma-derived growth factor)	AREG	21 (15.8 - 26.0)	0.055
coagulation factor III (thromboplastin, tissue factor)	F3	84 (37.7 - 131.1)	0.030
discs, large homolog 5 (Drosophila)	DLG5	13 (8.5 - 17.6)	0.114
interleukin 18 (interferon-gamma-inducing factor)	IL18	489 (146.4 - 831.2)	0.044
laminin, alpha 5	LAMA5	15 (8.8 - 20.4)	0.082
macrophage stimulating 1 receptor	MST1R	10 (8.2 - 12.8)	0.058
neuromedin U	NMU	311 (136.6 - 486.2)	0.103
protein kinase C, iota	PRKCI	4 (3.3 - 4.2)	0.037
retinoid X receptor, alpha	RXRA	13 (7.3 - 18.0)	0.075
ryanodine receptor 1 (skeletal)	RYR1	20 (15.9 - 25.1)	0.031
secreted and transmembrane 1	SECTM1	33 (12.4 - 53.2)	0.062
sema domain, immunoglobulin domain (Ig), short basic domain, secreted, (semaphorin) 3F	SEMA3F	4 (3.3 - 4.9)	0.015
Transcription Regulator Activity			
E74-like factor 4 (ets domain transcription factor)	ELF4	24 (6.2 - 41.4)	0.070
homeo box A9	HOXA9	45 (36.7 - 52.9)	0.007
Kruppel-like factor 4 (gut)	KLF4	9 (4.3 - 14.7)	0.011
Kruppel-like factor 5 (intestinal)	KLF5	36 (17.6 - 54.8)	0.073
retinoid X receptor, alpha	RXRA	13 (7.3 - 18.0)	0.075
tripartite motif-containing 29	TRIM29	372 (53.1 - 691.1)	0.065
Catalytic Activity			
adenosine kinase	ADK	6 (4.8 - 8.2)	0.086
aldehyde dehydrogenase 2 family (mitochondrial)	ALDH2	13 (8.1 - 18.8)	0.029
annexin A3	ANXA3	33 (16.2 - 49.2)	0.000
argininosuccinate synthetase	ASS	192 (124.7 - 259.0)	0.045
carbohydrate (chondroitin 6) sulfotransferase 3	CHST3	4 (2.9 - 5.8)	0.019
chromosome 9 open reading frame 3	C9orf3	21 (4.7 - 36.6)	0.051
creatine kinase, brain	CKB	8 (6.3 - 10.6)	0.031
cyclin-dependent kinase inhibitor 2A	CDKN2A	16 (11.0 - 20.6)	0.085
dual specificity phosphatase 1	DUSP1	7 (5.0 - 9.9)	0.067
GTP cyclohydrolase 1 (dopa-responsive dystonia)	GCH1	5 (3.9 - 6.7)	0.001
hypoxia-inducible factor prolyl 4-hydroxylase	PH-4	6 (4.1 - 8.1)	0.037
macrophage stimulating 1 receptor	MST1R	10 (8.2 - 12.8)	0.058
MCM4 minichromosome maintenance deficient 4	MCM4	4 (2.9 - 4.6)	0.036
phosphorylase kinase, beta	PHKB	3 (2.4 - 4.0)	0.014
phosphoserine phosphatase	PSPH	7 (4.8 - 9.7)	0.018
protein kinase C, iota	PRKCI	4 (3.3 - 4.2)	0.037
steroid-5-alpha-reductase, alpha polypeptide 1 delta 4-dehydrogenase alpha 1)	SRD5A1	3 (2.5 - 3.1)	0.006
zinc finger, BED domain containing 1	ZBED1	4 (2.3 - 5.0)	0.038
Binding Activity			
adenosine kinase	ADK	6 (4.8 - 8.2)	0.086
amphiregulin (schwannoma-derived growth factor)	AREG	21 (15.8 - 26.0)	0.055
annexin A3	ANXA3	33 (16.2 - 49.2)	0.000
annexin A8	ANXA8	33 (24.6 - 41.2)	0.076

argininosuccinate synthetase	ASS	192 (124.7 - 259.0)	0.045
discs, large homolog 5 (Drosophila)	DLG5	13 (8.5 - 17.6)	0.114
DnaJ (Hsp40) homolog, subfamily C, member 9	DNAJC9	3 (2.5 - 3.8)	0.055
E74-like factor 4 (ets domain transcription factor)	ELF4	24 (6.2 - 41.4)	0.070
F-box and leucine-rich repeat protein 11	FBXL11	4 (3.1 - 5.1)	0.025
fibulin 1	FBLN1	36 (11.1 - 60.4)	0.020
homeo box A9	HOXA9	45 (36.7 - 52.9)	0.007
hypoxia-inducible factor prolyl 4-hydroxylase	PH-4	6 (4.1 - 8.1)	0.037
interleukin 18 (interferon-gamma-inducing factor)	IL18	489 (146.4 - 831.2)	0.044
Kruppel-like factor 4 (gut)	KLF4	9 (4.3 - 14.7)	0.011
Kruppel-like factor 5 (intestinal)	KLF5	36 (17.6 - 54.8)	0.073
laminin, alpha 5	LAMA5	15 (8.8 - 20.4)	0.082
laminin, beta 3	LAMB3	13 (5.3 - 21.0)	0.015
macrophage stimulating 1 receptor	MST1R	10 (8.2 - 12.8)	0.058
MCM4 minichromosome maintenance deficient 4	MCM4	4 (2.9 - 4.6)	0.036
myosin VC	MYO5C	6 (5.1 - 7.5)	0.029
neuromedin U	NMU	311 (136.6 - 486.2)	0.103
PDZ domain containing 3	PDZK3	64 (21.2 - 106.2)	0.073
phosphorylase kinase, beta	PHKB	3 (2.4 - 4.0)	0.014
phosphoserine phosphatase	PSPH	7 (4.8 - 9.7)	0.018
plakophilin 3	PKP3	11 (7.2 - 14.4)	0.100
poly(A) binding protein interacting protein 1	PAIP1	3 (2.9 - 4.2)	0.004
protein kinase C, iota	PRKCI	4 (3.3 - 4.2)	0.037
related RAS viral (r-ras) oncogene homolog 2	RRAS2	4 (2.8 - 4.9)	0.001
retinoid X receptor, alpha	RXRA	13 (7.3 - 18.0)	0.075
ryanodine receptor 1 (skeletal)	RYR1	20 (15.9 - 25.1)	0.031
stratifin	SFN	54 (39.6 - 69.5)	0.082
THAP domain containing 10	THAP10	3 (2.6 - 3.8)	0.016
tripartite motif-containing 29	TRIM29	372 (53.1 - 691.1)	0.065
villin 2 (ezrin)	VIL2	3 (2.6 - 4.0)	0.037
zinc finger, BED domain containing 1	ZBED1	4 (2.3 - 5.0)	0.038
Enzyme Regulator Activity			
annexin A3	ANXA3	33 (16.2 - 49.2)	0.000
cyclin-dependent kinase inhibitor 2A	CDKN2A	16 (11.0 - 20.6)	0.085
phosphorylase kinase, beta	PHKB	3 (2.4 - 4.0)	0.014
PTPL1-associated RhoGAP 1	PARG1	13 (10.0 - 16.2)	0.004
secretory leukocyte protease inhibitor (antileukoproteinase)	SLPI	21 (16.1 - 26.7)	0.028
serine protease inhibitor, Kunitz type, 2	SPINT2	131 (91.8 - 169.7)	0.002
stratifin	SFN	54 (39.6 - 69.5)	0.082
Motor Activity			
myosin VC	MYO5C	6 (5.1 - 7.5)	0.029
Ras interacting protein 1	RASIP1	26 (17.6 - 35.1)	0.068
Structural Molecule Activity			
desmoplakin	DSP	54 (19.6 - 89.4)	0.104
fibulin 1	FBLN1	36 (11.1 - 60.4)	0.020
keratin 17	KRT17	70 (48.2 - 91.0)	0.040
keratin 18	KRT18	86 (2.1 - 170.6)	0.023
keratin 8	KRT8	42 (29.4 - 53.9)	0.034
laminin, alpha 5	LAMA5	15 (8.8 - 20.4)	0.082
laminin, beta 3	LAMB3	13 (5.3 - 21.0)	0.015
periplakin	PPL	168 (105.5 - 231.3)	0.068
plakophilin 3	PKP3	11 (7.2 - 14.4)	0.100

tuftelin 1	TUFT1	5 (4.6 - 5.8)	0.017
villin 2 (ezrin)	VIL2	3 (2.6 - 4.0)	0.037
Transporter Activity			
aldehyde dehydrogenase 2 family (mitochondrial)	ALDH2	13 (8.1 - 18.8)	0.029
laminin, beta 3	LAMB3	13 (5.3 - 21.0)	0.015
ryanodine receptor 1 (skeletal)	RYR1	20 (15.9 - 25.1)	0.031
solute carrier family 16, member 5	SLC16A5	19 (4.5 - 34.5)	0.082
solute carrier family 29 (nucleoside transporters), member 3	SLC29A3	10 (6.8 - 12.9)	0.027
solute carrier family 38, member 1	SLC38A1	75 (20.7 - 130.3)	0.007
solute carrier family 38, member 2	SLC38A2	3 (2.1 - 4.5	0.010
steroid-5-alpha-reductase, alpha polypeptide 1	SRD5A1	3 (2.5 - 3.1)	0.006
No Classification			
brain abundant, membrane attached signal protein 1	BASP1	196 (139.6 - 252.1)	0.065
CD24 antigen (small cell lung carcinoma cluster 4 antigen)	CD24	1308 (766 - 1850.8)	0.010
chromosome 19 open reading frame 21	C19orf21	7 (4.2 - 9.5)	0.004
chromosome 2 open reading frame 26	C2orf26	6 (4.2 - 7.2)	0.102
COBL-like 1	COBLL1	6 (3.8 - 7.5)	0.108
EPS8-like 2	EPS8L2	73 (43.7 - 103.0)	0.066
GTP cyclohydrolase 1 (dopa-responsive dystonia)	GCH1	5 (3.9 - 6.7)	0.001
hypothetical protein FLJ14054	FLJ14054	15 (12.6 - 17.9)	0.014
hypothetical protein FLJ20364	FLJ20364	3 (2.7 - 3.5)	0.000
hypothetical protein FLJ21918	FLJ21918	16 (10.3 - 22.2)	0.053
hypothetical protein FLJ22662	FLJ22662	14 (7.4 - 20.7)	0.067
inhibitor of DNA binding 1	ID1	32 (18.3 - 46.6)	0.013
inhibitor of DNA binding 2	ID2	3 (2.2 - 4.9)	0.001
KIAA0746 protein	KIAA0746	16 (6.7 - 26.4)	0.018
KIAA0947 protein	KIAA0947	4 (2.7 - 4.9)	0.044
neuroepithelial cell transforming gene 1	NET1	5 (4.9 - 6.0)	0.004
Nipped-B homolog (Drosophila)	NIPBL	4 (3.4 - 5.4)	0.016
podocalyxin-like	PODXL	9 (5.4 - 13.2)	0.002
programmed cell death 4 (neoplastic transformation inhibitor)	PDCD4	3 (2.6 - 3.8)	0.037
Rab6-interacting protein 2	ELKS	3 (2.4 - 3.2)	0.027
RelA-associated inhibitor	RAI	9 (6.5 - 12.4)	0.082
RNA-binding protein	FLJ20273	38 (20.0 -56.2)	0.030
RUN and SH3 domain containing 1	RUSC1	3 (2.3 - 2.9)	0.022
S-phase kinase-associated protein 2 (p45)	SKP2	7 (5.0 - 8.6)	0.100
tumor necrosis factor, alpha-induced protein 8	TNFAIP8	14 (9.4 - 18.5)	0.030
ubiquitously transcribed tetratricopeptide repeat, X chromosome	UTX	3 (2.7 - 3.8)	0.008

*) P-values calculated by T-test using normalised signals of the microarrays.
**) Fold Change calculated from the mean of the single fold changes of all 12 comparisons. Single fold changes were calculated from the Signal Log Ratios of the comparisons obtained from GeneChip Operating Software (Affymetrix).

Table 14. List and Classification of genes upregulated in melanocytic nevi with the V600E mutation of the *B-RAF* gene compared to nevi without *B-RAF* mutation.

Molecular Function/Gene Title	Gene Symbol	P-value*	Fold Change (95% CI)**
Protein Binding			
cadherin 19, type 2	CDH19	0.000	22.9 (15.1-30.7)
Rho-related BTB domain containing 3	RHOBTB3	0.000	10.4 (8.0-12.8)
pleiotrophin (heparin binding growth factor 8, neurite growth-promoting factor 1)	PTN	0.008	9.5 (8.0-10.9)
tumor necrosis factor receptor superfamily, member 11b (osteoprotegerin)	TNFRSF11B	0.000	8.6 (6.5-10.7)
S100 calcium binding protein, beta (neural)	S100B	0.002	6.9 (5.9-7.9)
adducin 3 (gamma)	ADD3	0.000	6.6 (5.3-8.0)
A disintegrin and metalloproteinase domain 23	ADAM23	0.000	6.6 (5.3-7.9)
Tyrosine 3-monooxygenase/tryptophan 5-monooxygenase activation protein, epsilon polypeptide	YWHAE	0.000	6.4 (5.4-7.4)
cyclin-dependent kinase inhibitor 2A (melanoma, p16, inhibits CDK4)	CDKN2A	0.197	5.9 (5.2-6.6)
fibroblast growth factor 2 (basic)	FGF2	0.000	5.9 (4.8-6.9)
deleted in liver cancer 1	DLC1	0.000	5.8 (5.0-6.7)
sarcoglycan, epsilon	SGCE	0.000	5.7 (4.7-6.8)
G protein-coupled receptor, family C, group 5, member B	GPRC5B	0.031	4.9 (4.3-5.5)
pirin (iron-binding nuclear protein)	PIR	0.010	4.7 (4.1-5.3)
platelet derived growth factor D	PDGFD	0.000	4.6 (4.1-5.2)
sin3-associated polypeptide, 30kDa	SAP30	0.000	4.1 (3.7-4.4)
heat shock 70kDa protein 8	HSPA8	0.000	4.1 (3.7-4.4)
neuroligin 1	NLGN1	0.000	4.1 (3.5-4.7)
B-cell translocation gene 1, anti-proliferative	BTG1	0.000	4.0 (3.6-4.5)
nuclear receptor subfamily 3, group C, member 1 (glucocorticoid receptor)	NR3C1	0.000	4.0 (3.6-4.4)
BH-protocadherin (brain-heart)	PCDH7	0.013	3.8 (3.6-4.0)
spondin 1, extracellular matrix protein	SPON1	0.000	3.8 (3.3-4.2)
ankyrin 2, neuronal	ANK2	0.000	3.7 (3.3-4.1)
A kinase (PRKA) anchor protein (gravin) 12	AKAP12	0.001	3.6 (3.2-3.9)
CD44 antigen (homing function and Indian blood group system)	CD44	0.012	3.1 (2.9-3.3)
nucleophosmin/nucleoplasmin, 3	NPM3	0.001	3.1 (2.8-3.3)
Catalytic Activity			
coagulation factor V (proaccelerin, labile factor)	F5	0.000	41.3 (14.7-67.8)
tripartite motif-containing 9	TRIM9	0.000	23.8 (16.0-31.7)
SWI/SNF related, matrix associated, actin dependent regulator of chromatin, subfamily a, member 1	SMARCA1	0.000	10.2 (6.2-14.1)
protease, serine, 23	PRSS23	0.001	7.1 (5.8-8.4)
phosphorylase, glycogen; liver (Hers disease, glycogen storage disease type VI)	PYGL	0.001	6.9 (5.7-8.1)
chromosome 11 open reading frame 8	C11orf8	0.000	6.6 (4.9-8.3)
UDP-Gal:betaGlcNAc beta 1,4- galactosyltransferase, polypeptide 6	B4GALT6	0.000	5.9 (4.3-7.5)
serum/glucocorticoid regulated kinase-like	SGKL	0.000	5.7 (4.5-7.0)
crystallin, lambda 1	CRYL1	0.024	5.6 (5.0-6.2)
hydroxyprostaglandin dehydrogenase 15-(NAD)	HPGD	0.000	4.7 (4.1-5.3)
protein phosphatase 1, regulatory (inhibitor) subunit 3C	PPP1R3C	0.001	4.6 (4.0-5.2)
dual specificity phosphatase 6	DUSP6	0.000	3.6 (3.3-4.0)
Guanine nucleotide binding protein (G protein), q polypeptide	GNAQ	0.000	3.5 (3.2-3.9)

SEC11-like 1 (S. cerevisiae)	SEC11L1	0.000	3.4 (3.1-3.8)
cytochrome c oxidase subunit VIIc	COX7C	0.000	3.3 (3.1-3.6)
cell growth regulator with ring finger domain 1	CGRRF1	0.000	2.9 (2.6-3.1)
Signal Transducer Activity			
glutamate receptor, ionotropic, AMPA 1	GRIA1	0.015	20.6 (14.1-27.1)
G protein-coupled receptor 37 (endothelin receptor type B-like)	GPR37	0.099	10.8 (9.6-11.9)
attractin-like 1	ATRNL1	0.001	7.4 (4.7-10.0)
nuclear receptor subfamily 0, group B, member 1	NR0B1	0.009	7.1 (5.6-8.6)
lipopolysaccharide-induced TNF factor	LITAF	0.000	3.4 (3.1-3.7)
Nucleic Acid Binding			
ets variant gene 1	ETV1	0.000	12.0 (8.6-15.4)
paternally expressed 10	PEG10	0.001	9.0 (7.1-10.9)
chromosome 10 open reading frame 56	C10orf56	0.000	5.1 (4.4-5.7)
forkhead box O1A (rhabdomyosarcoma)	FOXO1A	0.000	4.3 (3.7-4.8)
microphthalmia-associated transcription factor	MITF	0.000	4.2 (3.6-4.8)
CUG triplet repeat, RNA binding protein 2	CUGBP2	0.000	4.0 (3.5-4.5)
LSM8 homolog, U6 small nuclear RNA associated (S. cerevisiae)	LSM8	0.000	3.3 (3.0-3.5)
AT rich interactive domain 5B (MRF1-like)	ARID5B	0.000	3.0 (2.7-3.2)
Transporter Activity			
solute carrier family 16 (monocarboxylic acid transporters), member 4	SLC16A4	0.000	8.1 (6.4-9.8)
potassium inwardly-rectifying channel, subfamily J, member 13	KCNJ13	0.000	6.2 (4.8-7.6)
solute carrier family 6, member 15	SLC6A15	0.000	5.8 (5.0-6.5)
solute carrier family 39 (zinc transporter), member 6	SLC39A6	0.000	4.6 (4.0-5.2)
hypothetical protein DJ971N18.2	DJ971N18.2	0.000	3.5 (3.2-3.8)
Enzyme Regulator Activity			
serine (or cysteine) proteinase inhibitor, clade E (nexin, plasminogen activator inhibitor type 1), member 2	SERPINE2	0.070	7.7 (6.9-8.6)
development and differentiation enhancing factor 1	DDEF1	0.001	5.1 (4.3-5.8)
cyclin-dependent kinase inhibitor 1C (p57, Kip2)	CDKN1C	0.000	4.6 (3.9-5.2)
Structural Molecule Activity			
caveolin 1, caveolae protein, 22kDa	CAV1	0.000	4.4 (3.8- 5.0)
chromosome 15 open reading frame 15	C15orf15	0.000	3.6 (3.3-4.0)
No Classification			
scrapie responsive protein 1	SCRG1	0.000	15.3 (8.9-21.8)
KIAA0470	KIAA0470	0.000	11.7 (9.0-14.5)
angiopoietin-like 7	ANGPTL7	0.023	10.7 (7.2-14.3)
complement factor H	CFH	0.060	9.4 (7.4-11.4)
p53-regulated apoptosis-inducing protein 1	P53AIP1	0.001	8.9 (6.4-11.1)
complement factor H /// complement factor H-related 1	CFH /// CFHL1	0.013	8.8 (6.4-11.1)
cell adhesion molecule with homology to L1CAM (close homolog of L1)	CHL1	0.010	8.6 (6.8-10.4)
elongation of very long chain fatty acids (FEN1/Elo2, SUR4/Elo3, yeast)-like 2	ELOVL2	0.001	8.4 (6.4-10.4)
carcinoembryonic antigen-related cell adhesion molecule 1 (biliary glycoprotein)	CEACAM1	0.000	6.9 (5.2-8.6)
brain and acute leukemia, cytoplasmic	BAALC	0.000	6.8 (5.5-8.1)
hypothetical protein FLJ11017	FLJ11017	0.001	4.8 (4.1-5.5)

ankyrin repeat and SOCS box-containing 9	ASB9	0.001	4.7 (4.1-5.2)
oxysterol binding protein-like 8	OSBPL8	0.000	4.5 (3.8-5.2)
cyclin I	CCNI	0.000	4.4 (3.9-4.9)
pleckstrin and Sec7 domain containing 3	PSD3	0.000	4.4 (3.7-5.0)
Meis1, myeloid ecotropic viral integration site 1 homolog 4 (mouse)	MEIS4	0.000	4.2 (3.6-4.7)
AF034176 Human mRNA (Tripodis and Ragoussis) Homo sapiens cDNA clone ntcon5 contig	---	0.000	4.1 (3.7-4.6)
TM2 domain containing 1	TM2D1	0.000	4.0 (3.6-4.4)
microfibrillar-associated protein 3-like	MFAP3L	0.003	4.0 (3.5-4.5)
S-phase kinase-associated protein 1A (p19A)	SKP1A	0.000	3.7 (3.3-4.1)
cyclin G1	CCNG1	0.000	3.4 (3.1-3.7)
transmembrane protein 14B	TMEM14B	0.000	3.3 (3.0-3.6)
syntaxin binding protein 6 (amisyn)	STXBP6	0.002	3.2 (2.8-3.5)
sprouty homolog 2 (Drosophila)	SPRY2	0.000	3.1 (2.9-3.4)
chromosome 6 open reading frame 48	C6orf48	0.007	3.1 (2.9-3.4)
sterile alpha motif domain containing 4	SAMD4	0.000	3.0 (2.8-3.3)
eukaryotic translation elongation factor 1 epsilon 1	EEF1E1	0.000	3.0 (2.8-3.2)
dilute suppressor	DSU	0.001	2.8 (2.6-3.0)

Table 15. List and Classification of genes downregulated in melanocytic nevi with the V600E mutation of the *B-RAF* gene compared to nevi without *B-RAF* mutation.

Molecular Function/Gene Title	Gene Symbol	P-value*	Fold Change (95% CI)**
Nucleic Acid Binding			
FOS-like antigen 2	FOSL2	0.005	5.7 (4.4-7.0)
hairless homolog (mouse)	HR	0.011	4.4 (3.7-5.2)
cleavage and polyadenylation specific factor 1, 160kDa	CPSF1	0.073	4.4 (3.4-5.4)
DiGeorge syndrome critical region gene 8	DGCR8	0.042	4.3 (3.6-5.0)
GLI-Kruppel family member HKR3	HKR3	0.000	4.1 (0.4-7.8)
general transcription factor IIIC, polypeptide 1, alpha 220kDa	GTF3C1	0.003	4.0 (3.7-4.4)
HLA-B associated transcript 1	BAT1	0.006	3.9 (3.2-4.6)
A kinase (PRKA) anchor protein 8-like	AKAP8L	0.007	3.4 (3.1-3.7)
Protein Binding			
tropomyosin 2 (beta)	TPM2	0.241	13.4 (6.8-20.1)
lecithin-cholesterol acyltransferase	LCAT	0.019	9.6 (7.2-12.0)
chemokine (C-C motif) ligand 14 /// chemokine (C-C motif) ligand 15	CCL14 /// CCL15	0.024	6.7 (5.9-7.6)
Duffy blood group	FY	0.040	5.4 (3.5-7.3)
SIN3 homolog B, transcription regulator (yeast)	SIN3B	0.000	5.1 (4.6-5.6)
collagen, type VII, alpha 1 (epidermolysis bullosa, dystrophic, dominant and recessive)	COL7A1	0.034	5.0 (4.3-5.7)
collagen, type XVIII, alpha 1	COL18A1	0.001	4.9 (4.7-5.2)
rabaptin, RAB GTPase binding effector protein 2	RABEP2	0.000	4.8 (4.5-5.1)
thyroid hormone receptor associated protein 5	THRAP5	0.001	4.5 (4.0-5.0)
growth arrest-specific 6	GAS6	0.001	4.3 (3.9-4.7)
transgelin	TAGLN	0.234	4.2 (-0.9-9.2)
integrin, beta 4	ITGB4	0.000	4.1 (3.8-4.4)
tumor necrosis factor receptor superfamily, member 25	TNFRSF25	0.015	4.1 (-0.7-9.0)
Spectrin, alpha, non-erythrocytic 1 (alpha-fodrin)	SPTAN1	0.000	4.0 (2.7-5.4)
tumor necrosis factor receptor superfamily, member 25 /// pleckstrin homology domain containing, family G (with RhoGef domain) member 5	TNFRSF25 /// PLEKHG5	0.035	4.0 (0.6-7.4)
apolipoprotein E	APOE	0.078	3.9 (3.5-4.2)
euchromatic histone-lysine N-methyltransferase 2	EHMT2	0.017	3.9 (3.1-4.8)
FAT tumor suppressor homolog 2 (Drosophila)	FAT2	0.012	3.8 (3.3-4.2)
NACHT, leucine rich repeat and PYD containing 1	NALP1	0.064	3.7 (3.4-4.0)
tubulin-specific chaperone d	TBCD	0.009	3.6 (3.4-3.8)
type 1 tumor necrosis factor receptor shedding aminopeptidase regulator	ARTS-1	0.002	3.6 (3.1-4.0)
collagen, type VI, alpha 2	COL6A2	0.070	3.6 (2.0-5.2)
presenilin enhancer 2 homolog (C. elegans) /// protein F25965	PSENEN /// F25965	0.018	3.5 (3.0-4.0)
leucine-rich repeats and death domain containing	LRDD	0.000	3.5 (2.4-4.7)
adaptor-related protein complex 1, gamma 2 subunit	AP1G2	0.010	3.4 (3.2-3.7)
filamin A, alpha (actin binding protein 280)	FLNA	0.030	3.4 (2.6-4.2)
laminin, alpha 5	LAMA5	0.022	3.3 (2.9-3.7)
v-Ha-ras Harvey rat sarcoma viral oncogene homolog	HRAS	0.000	3.3 (2.9-3.7)
capping protein (actin filament), gelsolin-like	CAPG	0.058	3.3 (2.7-3.9)
glycoprotein Ib (platelet), beta polypeptide	GP1BB	0.013	3.3 (2.2-4.4)
endothelial cell growth factor 1 (platelet-derived)	ECGF1	0.131	3.2 (2.2-4.2)
sodium channel, nonvoltage-gated 1 alpha	SCNN1A	0.067	2.7 (2.3-3.1)

Enzyme Regulator Activity			
tyrosine kinase, non-receptor, 2	TNK2	0.006	5.0 (4.5-5.5)
MCF.2 cell line derived transforming sequence-like	MCF2L	0.031	4.6 (2.4-6.8)
TBC1 domain family, member 3 /// TBC1 domain family, member 3C	TBC1D3 /// TBC1D3C	0.013	4.5 (4.0-5.1)
serine (or cysteine) proteinase inhibitor, clade F (alpha-2 antiplasmin, pigment epithelium derived factor), member 1	SERPINF1	0.078	4.4 (3.6-5.3)
Rap guanine nucleotide exchange factor (GEF)-like 1	RAPGEFL1	0.007	3.8 (1.5-6.2)
misshapen-like kinase 1 (zebrafish)	MINK1	0.010	3.4 (2.9-3.9)
Ran GTPase activating protein 1	RANGAP1	0.007	3.1 (2.8-3.3)
Structural Molecule Activity			
keratin, hair, acidic, 1	KRTHA1	0.041	8.3 (6.0-10.5)
wingless-type MMTV integration site family, member 4	WNT4	0.024	4.4 (3.9-4.9)
envoplakin	EVPL	0.000	3.8 (2.4-5.1)
Catalytic Activity			
EPH receptor B6	EPHB6	0.001	9.1 (8.6-9.6)
matrix metalloproteinase 28	MMP28	0.004	8.1 (7.3-8.9)
phospholipase A2, group IVB (cytosolic)	PLA2G4B	0.002	7.0 (6.6-7.3)
HECT domain containing 3	HECTD3	0.010	6.4 (6.1-6.8)
cytochrome P450, family 3, subfamily A, polypeptide 5	CYP3A5	0.036	6.0 (5.5-6.6)
cyclin-dependent kinase (CDC2-like) 10	CDK10	0.007	6.0 (5.2-6.7)
KIAA0657 protein	KIAA0657	0.009	5.4 (4.9-5.8)
cytochrome P450, family 4, subfamily F, polypeptide 12	CYP4F12	0.025	5.1 (4.8-5.4)
carbonic anhydrase XII	CA12	0.037	5.1 (4.6-5.6)
proline dehydrogenase (oxidase) 1	PRODH	0.006	4.6 (3.9-5.3)
dual oxidase 1	DUOX1	0.012	4.1 (3.3-4.9)
choline kinase beta /// carnitine palmitoyltransferase 1B (muscle)	CHKB /// CPT1B	0.053	4.0 (2.9-5.1)
hyaluronoglucosaminidase 1	HYAL1	0.010	3.9 (3.6-4.2)
macrophage stimulating 1 receptor (c-met-related tyrosine kinase)	MST1R	0.000	3.7 (3.3-4.0)
diacylglycerol kinase, alpha 80kDa	DGKA	0.004	3.6 (3.0-4.1)
potassium voltage-gated channel, shaker-related subfamily, beta member 2	KCNAB2	0.098	3.6 (2.7-4.5)
ubiquitin-activating enzyme E1 (A1S9T and BN75 temperature sensitivity complementing)	UBE1	0.057	3.5 (2.8-4.1)
KIAA0220-like protein /// PI-3-kinase-related kinase SMG-1-like /// hypothetical protein 348162 /// hypothetica protein LOC440354	LOC23117 /// DKFZp547E087 /// LOC348162 /// LOC440354	0.020	3.4 (2.8-3.9)
amiloride binding protein 1 (amine oxidase (copper-containing))	ABP1	0.000	3.4 (2.0-4.8)
aldehyde dehydrogenase 3 family, memberA1	ALDH3A1	0.015	3.3 (2.7-3.8)
pyruvate kinase, muscle	PKM2	0.094	3.3 (1.9-4.8)
testis-specific kinase 1	TESK1	0.011	3.2 (2.9-3.4)
related RAS viral (r-ras) oncogene homolog	RRAS	0.018	3.0 (2.7-3.4)
tissue specific transplantation antigen P35B	TSTA3	0.000	2.9 (2.6-3.2)
Signal Transducer Activity			
jagged 2	JAG2	0.004	5.2 (4.8-5.6)
gamma-aminobutyric acid (GABA) A receptor, epsilon	GABRE	0.043	5.0 (4.1-5.8)
leukotriene B4 receptor	LTB4R	0.075	4.1 (3.1-5.2)
chromosome 8 open reading frame 20	C8orf20	0.002	3.9 (3.6-4.1)
gamma-aminobutyric acid (GABA) B receptor, 1	GABBR1	0.006	3.9 (3.5-4.3)

No Classification			
neuropathy target esterase	NTE	0.072	14.2 (13.7-14.0)
secretoglobin, family 1D, member 2	SCGB1D2	0.163	11.0 (3.5-18.6)
phospholipid transfer protein	PLTP	0.063	6.1 (5.6-6.6)
signal-transducing adaptor protein-2	STAP2	0.001	5.9 (5.6-6.3)
CD207 antigen, langerin	CD207	0.050	5.8 (4.8-6.9)
nuclear pore complex interacting protein /// hypothetical protein LOC339047 /// similar to hypothetical protein LOC339047	NPIP /// LOC339047 /// LOC440341	0.006	5.7 (5.3-6.1)
heat shock 27kDa protein 1	HSPB1	0.103	5.5 (4.3-6.7)
LRP16 protein	LRP16	0.001	5.2 (4.9-5.4)
up-regulated gene 4	URG4	0.000	4.7 (4.4-4.9)
protocadherin 21	PCDH21	0.007	4.6 (4.0-5.2)
CUB domain containing protein 1	CDCP1	0.009	4.5 (4.2-4.9)
hypothetical protein LOC339047	LOC339047	0.003	4.5 (4.1-4.9)
LOC399491 protein	LOC399491	0.010	4.4 (4.1-4.7)
hypothetical protein FLJ12681	FLJ12681	0.000	4.2 (3.9-4.6)
hypothetical protein FLJ22531	FLJ22531	0.010	4.0 (3.7-4.3)
protein tyrosine phosphatase, receptor type, f polypeptide (PTPRF), interacting protein (liprin), alpha 3	PPFIA3	0.000	4.0 (3.7-4.2)
myeloid leukemia factor 2	MLF2	0.051	4.0 (3.6-4.5)
Fc fragment of IgG binding protein	FCGBP	0.075	3.8 (3.5-4.2)
Ras interacting protein 1	RASIP1	0.072	3.7 (3.0-4.4)
CDC20 cell division cycle 20 homolog (S. cerevisiae)	CDC20	0.023	3.7 (2.7-4.7)
sema domain, immunoglobulin domain (Ig), short basic domain, secreted, (semaphorin) 3F	SEMA3F	0.002	3.6 (3.3-4.0)
uncoupling protein 2 (mitochondrial, proton carrier)	UCP2	0.062	3.6 (3.0-4.3)
carcinoembryonic antigen-related cell adhesion molecule 6 (non-specific cross reacting antigen)	CEACAM6	0.161	3.5 (3.0-4.0)
T-cell, immune regulator 1, ATPase, H+ transporting, lysosomal V0 protein a isoform 3	TCIRG1	0.008	3.4 (2.3-4.4)

*) P-values calculated by T-test using normalised signals of the microarrays
**) Fold Change calculated from the mean of the single fold changes of all 72 comparisons. Single fold changes were calculated from the Signal Log Ratios of the comparisons obtained from Data Mining Tool (Affymetrix).

9. OWN PUBLICATIONS

1. Bloethner, S., Chen, B., Hemminki, K., Mueller-Berghaus, J., Ugurel, S., Schadendorf, D. and Kumar, R. (2005) Effect of common *B-RAF* and *N-RAS* mutations on global gene expression in melanoma cell lines. *Carcinogenesis,* **26,** 1224-32.

2. Bloethner, S., Hemminki, K., Thirumaran, R. K., Chen, B., Mueller-Berghaus, J., Ugurel, S., Schadendorf, D. and Kumar, R (2005) Differences in global gene expression in melanoma cell lines with and without homozygous deletion of the *CDKN2A* locus genes. *Melanoma Res,* manuscript (revised version) submitted

3. Ugurel, S., Thirumaran, R. K., Bloethner, S., Gast, A., Sucker, A., Mueller Berghaus, J., Rittgen, W., Hemminki, K., Kumar, R. and Schadendorf, D (2005) Differential prognostic impact of the mutational status of *B-RAF* and *N-RAS* in melanoma. *J Clin Oncol,* manuscript submitted

4. Bloethner, S., Gast, A., Snellman, E., Thirumaran, R., Angelini, S., Hemminki, K and Kumar, R (2005) Effect of the V600E *B-RAF* mutation on global gene expression in benign melanocytic nevi. Manuscript in preparation

5. Bloethner, S., Ugurel, S., Chen, B., Mueller-Berghaus, J., Schadendorf, D., Hemminki, K. and Kumar, R (2005) Quantification of B-RAF, N-RAS and CDKN2A gene expression in metastatic melanoma cell lines. Manuscript in preparation

10. ACKNOWLEDGEMENTS

The studies described in this thesis have been carried out at the Department of Molecular-Genetic Epidemiology, German Cancer Research Center, Heidelberg, Germany. I would like to express my sincere gratitude to all who have helped and supported me during these three years. Especially I would like to thank:

Professor Kari Hemminki, for giving me the opportunity to work in a modern, creative and highly stimulating research environment with a unique international touch.

Associate professor Rajiv Kumar, my doctoral supervisor, for suggesting my PhD project and for introducing me to the field of melanoma. I am grateful for giving me the opportunity to work on "expression" and for his trust. His great enthusiasm, immediate advice and help in bringing up new ideas were very supporting and pushed me forward in critical moments.

Professor Claus R. Bartram, my advisor at the Medical Faculty of the Ruprecht-Karls-University of Heidelberg, for his support.

Professor Dirk Schadendorf and PD Dr. Selma Ugurel, for a very pleasant and fruitful cooperation, for providing excellent and valuable cell and tissue material, for giving interesting insights into the clinical side of our research and for helpful discussions and advice.

Dr. Wieland Keilholz, the Affymetrix field application specialist, for his great and patient support throughout those three years in everything connected to "Affymetrix" and for immediately being on the spot in "emergency" cases.

All my co-authors for their valuable contribution to the work.

All the participating melanoma patients and their families, without whom this work would never have been possible.

My PhD student colleagues in the "first room": Michael Wirtenberger, Kerstin Wagner, Ranjit K. Thirumaran and Kalai S. Shanmugam, for interesting conversations and discussions and even for sharing silence sometimes.

All my other colleagues and friends in the group: Justo Lorenzo Bermejo, Dagmar Beisse, Andrea Altieri, Andreas Gast, Eva Hiripi, Felipe Castro, Sonali Chandra, Bernd Frank, Barbara Burwinkel, Asta Försti, Annika Vaclavicek, Stefan Wilkening, Julia Schmutzhard, Marion Gangel-Drechsel, Bowang Chen, Sandrine Tchatchou, Haixin Lei and Xuchen Li for a pleasant and supporting work environment, interesting conversations and a unique international athmosphere in the lab.

Bowang Chen, Justo Lorenzo Bermejo and Eva Hiripi for help in handling the crowd of "Affy data" and other statistical analyses.

My close friends outside (and inside) the laboratory, for support, nice conversations, pleasant afternoons at the "Neckarwiese" and all the activities which made my time in Heidelberg unforgettable.

My friends outside Heidelberg, for fantastic emails, endless phone calls and visits. You all gave me big encouragement and support, even though you were far away!

My family: Special thanks goes to my mother, Brigitte, for the steady love, support and encouragement throughout my whole education time. Furthermore, I thank my sister Corinna, my uncle Reinhard and my aunt Kerstin for love and support and for encouraging me in my decisions; especially for the patient and immediate help when I again had to carry my furniture from one flat to another.

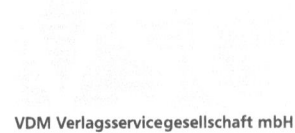

VDM Verlagsservicegesellschaft mbH

Die VDM Verlagsservicegesellschaft sucht für wissenschaftliche Verlage abgeschlossene und herausragende

Dissertationen, Habilitationen, Diplomarbeiten, Master Theses, Magisterarbeiten usw.

für die kostenlose Publikation als Fachbuch.

Sie verfügen über eine Arbeit, die hohen inhaltlichen und formalen Ansprüchen genügt, und haben Interesse an einer honorarvergüteten Publikation?

Dann senden Sie bitte erste Informationen über sich und Ihre Arbeit per Email an *info@vdm-vsg.de*.

Sie erhalten kurzfristig unser Feedback!

VDM Verlagsservicegesellschaft mbH
Dudweiler Landstr. 99
D - 66123 Saarbrücken
Telefon +49 681 3720 174
Fax +49 681 3720 1749

www.vdm-vsg.de

Die VDM Verlagsservicegesellschaft mbH vertritt

 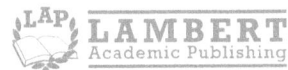 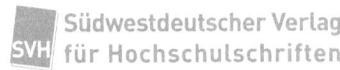

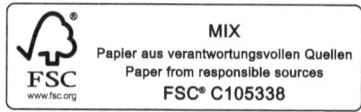

Printed by Books on Demand GmbH, Norderstedt / Germany